COMMON SENSE ABOUT YOGA

SONYA RICHMOND

Common Sense about Yoga

MacGibbon & Kee London

Granada Publishing Limited
First published in Great Britain 1971 by MacGibbon & Kee Ltd
3 Upper James Street London WIR 4BP

Copyright © 1971 by Sonya Richmond

ISBN 0 261 63235 3
Printed in Great Britain by The Barleyman Press, Bristol

TO MY TEACHER AND MY PUPILS

ACKNOWLEDGEMENTS

I wish to tender grateful acknowledgement to Methuen and Co. Ltd, London, for permission to quote passages translated by Juan Mascaró in his anthology *Lamps of Fire*.

I also wish to acknowledge my indebtedness to the late Swami Swarupananda whose rendering of the Bhagavad Gita has been, of the many I have studied, a particular source of inspiration and insight.

S.R.

CONTENTS

INTRODUCTION

With the sword of the understanding of thyself thou shalt rend asunder in thy heart every doubt arising from ignorance, and thou shalt achieve thy permanence in Yoga.

The Bhagavad Gita

THOSE of my readers who have read my book, *Yoga and Your Health*, will know the above quotation because I chose it to conclude the book. Now I choose it again to begin the present book because it is, because it always will be, one of the most succinct explanations of what this vast subject is all about.

Yoga is here to stay in the Western world. There can be little doubt about that. It is more popular in Western Europe and the United States than at any time in its three thousand year old history. But it would be difficult, if not impossible, to name a subject which has given rise to more fallacies and misconceptions, about which more incredible nonsense is written and spoken and believed, and whose fundamental aims are less understood than this timeless, down-to-earth philosophy.

I have long listened to these improbable results of muddled thinking, seen otherwise intelligent people with their minds locked and barred against Yoga because of the few undigested facts at their disposal; I have patiently told hundreds of enquirers, 'No, I do not sleep on a bed of nails—they would be so uncomfortable,' and 'No, I do not stand around on my head all day long, I have my husband and my home to look after, my books to write, my pupils to teach.' I have answered the most unbelievable questions with a straight face but still people go on believing the fallacies and not the facts about Yoga.

Exercising patience in the teeth of all this has been very good discipline for me, but has not gone very far in helping people to see Yoga in its true light, and I have long known that one day I would have to write a book called *Common Sense About Yoga*. Here it is.

SONYA RICHMOND

Ancora imparo—Still I am learning

Said to be a favourite motto of Michelangelo

Chapter 1

FACTS AND FALLACIES ABOUT YOGA

I feel myself, and I daresay that you have the same feeling, how hard is the attainment of any certainty about questions such as these in the present life. And yet I should regard a man as a coward who did not test what is said about them to the uttermost, or whose heart failed him before he had examined them on every side. For he should persevere until he has achieved one of two things: either he should discover the truth about them for himself, or learn it from others: or, if this be impossible, I would have him take the best and most irrefragable of human theories, and let this be the raft upon which he sails through life ...

PLATO *Phaedo*
From the translation by Jowett

1. *What exactly is Yoga?*

Many books have been written about Yoga, both in India and the West, but few of them explain, in a manner that the average reader can understand, exactly what it is. Consequently many people have an entirely mistaken idea as to what to expect when they decide to study Yoga and are lucky enough to find a Yoga teacher.

Some people think it is merely a means of relaxation. Some think it is an infallible cure for every known ailment. Some think it involves nothing but sitting in the lotus posture in a state of meditation, or standing on one's head for half an hour every morning. Most people who know nothing at all about it think there is some secret about it which will give them superiority over their fellow men. The unkindest ones dismiss it as some kind of cult for cranks but never bother to take any steps to find out whether they are right or wrong about this.

So what exactly *is* Yoga? First let us look in an English dictionary and here discover that 'Yoga is an ancient Hindu system of philosophic meditation and asceticism designed to effect the reunion of the devotee's soul with the Universal Spirit'. The Indian dictionaries are scarcely more helpful. We read something like 'Yoga is a method by which one can remove manifoldness and thus attain union with the Supreme Self'.

What does all this mean, in plain English? Technically Yoga refers to a system of philosophy propounded by an Indian sage, Patanjali, who lived about the second century B.C. His aphorisms enunciate the laws and principles of controlling the mind and teach how to translate these into action so that man's lower or bodily self becomes unified with his higher or spiritual self. This spiritual self the Hindus call the Atman which may be defined as perfect equilibrium between the body and the soul, or as the divine spark which the Hindus believe is in every individual. Through four Yogas it is possible to attain perfect physical health and moral and spiritual perfection.

Many of my readers will wonder why I chose to head this chapter with a quotation from a Greek instead of a Hindu philosopher. It is simply this: that the truths of Yoga are not confined to Hindu philosophy and that great thinkers from all over the world have arrived at the conclusions to be found in the great books of India. Compare, for instance, these two quotations:

The body is like the mortal and the soul is like the Divine.

PLATO

These bodies are perishable, but the dwellers in these bodies are eternal, indestructible and impenetrable.

The Bhagavad Gita

Plato leads men to the realm of ideas, and his great pupil Aristotle directed them to the study of nature. Plato made reason the basis of knowledge, Aristotle gave this place to experience. Though Aristotle is known as 'The Father of Logic', an equally developed system of logic existed at least two centuries before him, founded by Gautama, who is the author of the Nyaya system of Hindu philosophy, or Indian Logic. It is agreed generally by scholars of the two that each man evolved his system independently.

Let me sum up my answer to the question: What is Yoga? by a comparison of quotations from two other intellectual giants, both noted for their common sense approach to life and its problems—

Swami Vivekananda, the great Hindu Yoga teacher, orator and philosopher, and Schopenhauer, the German philosopher.

People prefer to be assured that life is sweetness and light. If we accept the premise that pain is the positive element of existence, this would seem to be a more realistic approach.

SCHOPENHAUER

Life is the unfoldment and development of a being under circumstances tending to press it down.

SWAMI VIVEKANANDA

The whole of this process forms the scope of Yoga.

2. *Yoga succeeds where medicine fails, does it not?*

Yoga and medicine are not mutually exclusive, though the method of approach to the patient in each case is different. Many of my pupils have been doctors and I have learned from them and they have learned from Yoga. Generally speaking in Yoga the psychological aspects of disease are given more attention than in the case of medicine. Yoga teachers prefer to investigate underlying causes of physical and emotional disorder rather than just treat the symptoms. Doctors usually use drugs or surgery to effect cures, whereas Yoga teachers will not advise their use unless absolutely necessary. Common sense is the keynote here. No Yoga teacher can cure appendicitis, for instance, and if an operation is not performed (and quickly!) the patient will suffer intolerable pain and ultimately die.

On the other hand, Yoga methods have spectacular success in such cases as overweight, underweight, many respiratory infections including asthma, sinus troubles and bronchitis, and in the treatment of psychological and emotional disorders including migraine, nervous tension, depression, insomnia, and the various neuroses. Yoga cannot, any more than medicine can, renew worn or damaged tissues. Spare-part surgery is entirely within the province of medicine in cases where it is applicable and is therefore outside the scope of this book.

To conclude, it is a known fact that in those cases which can be treated equally well by Yoga or medicine, some patients respond more readily to the Yoga method than to medicine and vice versa.

3. *Is it true that people who practise Yoga never grow old?*

I am always being asked this question and, once more, common sense is the answer. If it were in fact true, the word would certainly have got about in the three thousand years that Yoga has been put down systematically in writing, and Man would have solved one of the major problems of life. There would be no old people to be seen. So let us be logical about this.

No form of Yoga interferes with the natural processes of the body and the mind. Ageing is a natural process and not even Yoga can turn back the clock or halt the wear and tear of time. What Yoga *can* do is to prolong youth, that is the vitality and the active life of the individual, often well into middle age and even beyond. Also, if practised systematically and regularly, Yoga can prevent senility, and very elderly people can often retain their mental faculties until the end of life. I feel bound to say, though, that these benefits are by no means unknown in people who never practise Yoga at all but this is, perhaps, fortuitous. The practice of Yoga *ensures* that the benefits will accrue, leaving out the element of chance.

4. *How does Yoga influence intelligence?*

Yogis believe that there is no limit to the achievement of those who have mastered the combination of the three disciplines, asana (posture), pranayama (control of the breath), and developing the constructive power of the mind.

The Western attitude to the measurement of intelligence can be described as follows. Intelligence tests are not based on any specially sound scientific principles, and there is little agreement among psychologists as to the nature of intelligence itself. However, despite the arguments which still go on over this controversial subject, there is no doubt that intelligence tests have been outstandingly successful in their practical application.

Psychology is the offspring of philosophy and physiology. Philosophers, including Yogis, have always been interested in the cognitive powers of the mind. As late as 1904 the French psychologist, Binet, for the purpose of measuring relative intelligence, devised a series of thirty problems or tests calling for judgement, comprehension and reasoning, the problems being of such a nature that they could be understood without the benefit of any kind of special learning.

The measurement of intelligence has remained, despite its many imperfections, very popular. There is no doubt, for instance, that some people have an aptitude for passing I.Q. tests (as others have for chess, crossword puzzles, anagrams, bridge etc.) and therefore score higher marks than would otherwise be the case. But for the purposes of answering the above question these need not be taken into account. What remains to be examined is the terminal age and it is generally agreed by psychologists that by the time a person has reached physical maturity his intellectual ability has stabilized to a considerable extent and is not likely to change.

Yoga in no way accepts this view and there are many people in the world whose intelligence is both far above average and far above what it was at their age of physical maturity as a direct result of the practice of Yoga. It has been proved conclusively by Yoga teachers over the centuries that the Yoga techniques for the development of the intellect far beyond what psychologists call the terminal age, are and always have been entirely successful through the study of Raja or Jnana Yoga. These Yogas teach one to think logically and to use the intellect at all times to its utmost capacity so that one ultimately reaches one's full intellectual potential.

5. *What is the Vedanta?*

Think of a triangle. One side is the philosophy of Yoga, the other is the recognition of a higher, unseen controlling power, with the morality connected therewith. This is universally known as religion, and where religion and philosophy meet, at the apex of the triangle, there is the Vedanta.

To the sages of ancient India this was known as the Sanatana Dharma, the perennial philosophy or the Eternal Religion, and the findings of the Vedanta form the philosophical basis for a system of metaphysics which fulfils reason and gives Man the theoretical knowledge of the true nature of the universe and also provides the techniques by means of which he can realize this knowledge.

The philosophy of the Vedanta evolved from the Upanishads, one of the sections of the Vedas, which forms, with one or two exceptions, the concluding chapters of these most sacred scriptures of the Hindus.

The Vedanta is essentially pantheistic, demonstrating as it does the essential unity of all religions. Sri Ramakrishna, the great Bengali saint, put it succinctly when he uttered the now famous words: 'As many faiths, so many paths.' The Vedanta accepts all the great spiritual leaders of the world as being manifestations of the one Godhead and because it accepts all religions as such, it has no need of converts. Indeed it helps one to clarify and strengthen one's own religious belief. It has three fundamental truths:

    1. That the essential nature (the Self) of Man is divine.

    2. That the true aim of human life is to realize this.

    3. That Truth is universal and not the exclusive monopoly of any one race, creed or epoch.

Sri Ramakrishna set out the right attitudes towards religious differences, and his sayings, some of which I will quote here, demonstrate the amazing broadmindedness of the man and the unusually tolerant nature of this timeless religion.

God is one but His aspects are many. As the master of a house is father to one, brother to another, and husband to a third, and is called by different names by different persons, so the one God is described in various ways according to the particular aspect in which He appears to His particular worshipper . . .

As a mother, in nursing her sick children, gives rice and curry to one, sago and arrowroot to another, and bread and butter to a third, so the Lord has laid out different paths for different men *suitable to their natures* . . .

A truly religious man should think that other religions are also so many paths leading to the Truth. We should always maintain an attitude of respect towards other religions.

All the great thinkers of the Vedanta were concerned with the Truth of things and a dispassionate study of life and experience in their totality. This search for the highest Truth together with an absorbing interest in human welfare and happiness has transformed a world-view into a social philosophy. The book that documents this philosophy is the Bhagavad Gita, and the meaning and scope of it is elucidated by Swami Vivekananda, the great pupil of Sri Ramakrishna, in the well-known statement of Vedantic faith:

Each soul is potentially divine. The goal is to manifest this Divinity within by controlling nature, external and internal. Do this either by work (Karma Yoga), or worship (Bhakti Yoga), mental control (Raja Yoga), or philosophy (Jnana Yoga), by one or more or all of these—and be free.

There is one rich word in Indian philosophy which expresses all the means by which Man can release the mind from its lower self and having realized the true Self, live life in the fullest possible sense. That word is Yoga.

6. *Why do the names of the Vedantist Monks end in the syllables Ananda?*
Ananda is the Sanskrit word for Bliss.

7. *What does Swami Vivekananda's name mean?*
A swami is a Hindu monk, and Vivekananda means philosophical discrimination and bliss.

8. *What is the Bhagavad Gita and what does the name mean?*
This is the beautiful and world-renowned Hindu scripture written in poetry, which comprises eighteen chapters of the epic Sanskrit poem, 'Mahabharata'. The Gita describes the upward struggle of a human soul from ignorance to the highest Knowledge. The name is translated as The Song of the Blessed One or the Song of God. As it is by far the most popular Hindu scripture I have devoted the whole of Chapter Two of this book to an analysis of it.

9. *What are the three Gunas mentioned in the Gita?*
According to the Gita, Nature or matter consists of three Gunas or qualities known as sattva, rajas, and tamas. Sattva means balance or righteousness, and is described in the Gita as luminous, shining and free from evil. Rajas means restlessness or activity and is described in the Gita as passion. Tamas means inertia or dullness and is described in the Gita as ignorance which stupefies all embodied beings. The Gunas are essentially rocks strewn across the path of Self-Awareness, because they bind the individual to the lower self. Sattva binds one to the idea of happiness, Rajas to action, and Tamas to

21

lack of comprehension. The idea in the Gita is that the individual should be aware of the three Gunas and not hate them but rise above them.

Lord Krishna refers to this idea in the following words:

When the seer beholds no agent other than the Gunas and knows that which is higher than the Gunas, he attains to My Being. The embodied one having gone beyond these three Gunas, out of which the body is evolved, is freed from birth, death, decay and pain, and attains to immortality.

10. *What is the meaning of Maya?*

Maya is said to consist of the three Gunas which are described as the three strands which form the rope by which Man is bound to the illusory world. Maya does not exist independently of the three Gunas. Maya is a term of Vedanta philosophy denoting the ignorance which obscures Reality.

11. *Is there any difference between the disciplines of the Vedanta and those of Yoga?*

Vedantic teachers recommend the Yoga system as set down by Patanjali as a *practical discipline* for the attainment of samadhi or that state in which true Knowledge is realized by the individual. There is very little difference between the Vedantic disciplines and the Yogic disciplines, the latter being the practical and scientific systematization of the spiritual disciplines prevalent in Patanjali's time.

12. *What is the meaning of the sound OM?*

In Indian philosophy the syllable OM represents the root of all articulate sound. It is the most sacred word of the Vedas and is also written AUM. It is a symbol of both the personal God and the Absolute, but it is more than a word of appellation. In Indian thought the syllable is a representation of the sound in which God is considered to be manifest and its repetition is recommended for the stilling of the mind's whirling thoughts, and the deflection of negative emotions.

For Western people the repetition of the sound OM (or AUM) possibly has the further advantage of neutrality without any anthropomorphic connotations, and therefore as a symbol it is doubly valuable.

13. *Does Yoga make any concessions to human fallibility?*

Believe it or not it does, though to read some of the books written on Yoga, one would hardly think so. But the Bhagavad Gita has many layers of meaning and is therefore open to different interpretations, and one of these can be on an entirely human level. At first reading the Gita is an esoteric poem of great beauty and wisdom but the Westerner, in particular, has difficulty in identifying himself with what appears to be a dialogue between God and a warrior Prince.

In actual fact it can be read as a dialogue between Everyman and his conscience. Arjuna/Everyman appears at the very beginning of the Gita as a human being with a problem. For the purposes of answering this question it does not matter what that problem is. What does matter is Arjuna's reaction to it which is the reaction of any ordinary person. He is so grieved and bewildered by his dilemma that his judgement is clouded to the extent that he is quite unable to find a solution. Does this not happen to all of us when first we are confronted with a problem? It is only by becoming objective, standing back a little, that we can see the problem in its true perspective, reduce it to its real size and thereby discover the solution in our own minds.

If we can therefore think of the god, Krishna, as Arjuna's conscience, then we can see that this man, in order to find the solution to his dilemma, turns his thoughts inwards. The great German philosopher, Kant, speaks of the 'moral law within' in his *Critique of Practical Reason* and some people consider that this inner moral law is, in fact, the divine spark in every human being. It does not seem to me that this argument is in any way far-fetched. The psyche is self-regulating and has an instinctive wisdom which is entirely autonomous. The name of Kant is applicable again here for it was he who formulated the doctrine that the human will carries its guiding principle within itself.

Man's growing sophistication has largely disconnected him from what may be termed 'nature's instinctive wisdom', but fortunately this process has not been completed otherwise Man would scarcely be able to survive. At moments of profound uncertainty, as is the case with Arjuna in the Gita, the instinct, when given the chance to operate, shows a knowledge of the underlying situation and the 'moral law within' is the means by which the psyche regulates itself to the benefit of the entire organism.

It is typical of an ordinary man's reaction, though, that the giving up of the wilful authority of the ego in favour of the moral law within produces a reaction of extreme reluctance—in other words, it seems easier to give in to panic and despair than to obey one's conscience. Listen to the words of Arjuna to Krishna (his conscience) when Krishna tells him that he must fight his own kinsmen because it is his duty to do so.

But, Krishna, if according to Thee knowledge is superior to action, why then do you urge me to do these terrible deeds? With these seemingly conflicting words, Thou art, as it were, bewildering my understanding.

And further on, still in a state of reluctance he says,

Krishna, what makes a man do evil, even when it is against his own *will*? It is as though he were constrained by force.

I have stressed the word will because the will and the ego are first cousins and once the ego gets the upper hand one cannot see the workings of one's own conscience. The psyche responds to our perception by uncovering a purpose which transcends personal wishes formed in ego-consciousness. It is this uncovering process which forms the subject matter of the Bhagavad Gita. Looked at in this way, and it is perfectly feasible to do so, the Gita is a very human book about a very human and fallible person. It is this very fact, I believe, that makes the Gita so wholly timeless and why in the 1970s it has so much to teach us. Perhaps we have never needed it more than we do in these troubled times.

14. *Does Yoga develop extra-sensory perception?*

I am often asked this and it is, of course, begging the question. Some people believe there is such a thing as E.S.P. and others do

24

not. Yoga's techniques aim towards the development of self-aware-ness and part of this process, as I mentioned in the answer to the preceding question, is the transcendence of ego-consciousness, the subjugation of one's personal wishes and desires. It follows natur-ally that if one is so far advanced in Yoga as to be able to do this, one can view a situation in its totality with one's judgement un-impaired by the ego, and logic will do the rest. It is possible that a person who has in his hands so infallible a weapon as logic would be able to predict situations far in advance of their happening or even be able to arrive at an awareness of their happening currently. As the ability to think with so high a degree of clarity and logic would only be possible to someone very advanced in Yoga, it would naturally appear to people generally that such a person was gifted with extra-sensory perception.

15. *Does one have to be a vegetarian to practise Yoga?*
In spite of what many Yoga books say about the eating of 'dead' foods, that is flesh foods, it does remain purely a matter of per-sonal choice. We are all different individuals and it is a medical fact that some people manage to keep perfectly healthy on a vege-tarian diet while others keep healthy on a diet which includes flesh foods, and in fact would not do so well on a vegetarian diet. I think that one should use common sense in this matter, though as a Yoga teacher I have met more food faddists and fanatical vege-tarians than I could possibly count. Yoga insists on a person not being fanatical about anything and it follows that it is against all the laws of Yoga to impose one's personal views, about diet or any-thing else, upon another person. The rule here would be to get to know your own needs so far as food is concerned and not sacrifice your health and well-being to a misplaced principle.

16. *Is Yoga slimming?*
This, of course, I am asked constantly. The grim business of losing weight is a subject about which more fallacies are pro-pounded than almost any other. To give a full and common sense answer, let us suppose that a person consistently overeats for ten, fifteen, twenty years, builds up a good thick layer of subcutaneous fat and is several stone overweight. Would such a person, by tak-

ing up the study and practice of Yoga, become slender without making any other effort?

Let us say it depends not only on what kind of Yoga but also on how far he is prepared to progress. Leaving aside Hatha Yoga (that is the physical discipline) for a moment, and supposing that our hypothetical person becomes interested in the philosophy of Yoga, what then? Theoretically any of the Yogas of the mind, if practised with diligence, would in time result in an expansion of intellectual awareness and things of the mind would gradually take precedence over those of the body. Also if he reads his Gita and practises what he reads, i.e. 'Success in Yoga is not for him who eats too much or too little, nor, O Arjuna, for him who sleeps too much or too little.'

The Yoga-shastra directs half of the stomach for food and condiments, a quarter for water and a quarter for the free motion of air. Such a regimen would almost certainly result in a considerable loss of fat in an overweight person. So our student would, by degrees, if he practised Yoga to the letter, grow disinclined to overeat. He would, in fact, be repelled by his bloated appearance which so blatantly demonstrated to the world that he was a person who over-indulged himself in the matter of food and took little exercise.

But let us be realistic. People who consistently overeat or who are compulsive eaters have a psychological problem and they, more than anyone else, need a Yoga teacher to do two things: find out the underlying cause of the overeating and secondly—and here is where common sense comes into it—to put the pupil on a sensible, balanced diet. So I would not recommend to Westerners any of the intellectual Yogas as a realistic slimming method. For one thing it would take too long to lose weight that way, but by far the more important factor is that few people could develop the degree of self-discipline involved. People are frail human beings. A piece of bad news, the loss of a job, pre-menstrual tension, a bereavement, any kind of adversity can send a man to the bottle and a woman to the chocolates or the cream cakes.

Now what of Hatha Yoga, the physical discipline? This subject I deal with in my book, *Yoga and Your Health*. I will deal briefly with it here. Hatha Yoga was devised as a system of physical postures and breathing exercises to bring the body to such a high degree of health that it can, as it were, be 'forgotten'. One is then free to develop the mind. This is sheer common sense because no one, not even a Yogi, could concentrate for very long on the higher things of the mind if he were plagued by migraine or indigestion, or any kind of physical discomfort. So one can achieve, by the practice of Hatha Yoga, superb health and greatly increased vitality and zest for life. But slimming? With Hatha Yoga one can say, yes, you can slim in due course by doing just Hatha Yoga and eating as much as you like. Because in time you would be less inclined to eat more than you need, for the fact is that any kind of Yoga, even the physical discipline, has an effect on the mental processes and one grows more moderate in all one's habits. In the Gita it says, 'He who is moderate in food and movements, in his actions and in sleep and wakefulness, attains to Yoga.' And the actual practice of any form of Yoga helps one towards this moderation.

But I do not believe there is any Yoga teacher who would teach Hatha Yoga to a pupil who was grossly overweight without suggesting he go on a sensible eating programme. And this so-called 'Yoga diet' works more effectively than any other that has ever been devised. Yoga is nothing if not common sense and so in the matter of working out a diet for a pupil, any teacher who was an expert in dietetics (and most Yoga teachers are), would start with psychology. Knowing that people who consistently overeat have a psychological dependence on food, and often sweet and starchy foods, the teacher's first question is likely to be, 'What food do you absolutely have to have when you are upset?' The answer, if it is a woman, is almost certain to be either chocolate, sweet cakes, biscuits or ice-cream. Men tend to prefer alcohol when upset, and that of course is high in calories and often carbohydrates as well and therefore fattening.

I have not the space in this book to explain the principles of the infallible Yoga diet, so let it suffice to say that, because it leans so heavily on the psychological needs and capabilities of the individual, each diet is worked out to suit the particular pupil in question, and if he (or she) has psychological dependence on a certain food, however fattening it may be it is incorporated into the diet. This is sound psychology. If you tell a person they cannot have this or that they will be disheartened before they start and the diet will not work. So a positive approach is the Yoga method. And while the pupil is allowed the food he most 'needs' in a crisis, the rest of the diet is so designed as to give him so much to eat that he will gradually feel the need lessen and finally disappear.

It takes a lot of psychology to get a fat woman off cream cakes or chocolates but Yoga teachers certainly know how it is done.

17. *What is the Atman?*

The determination of the nature of reality is the quest of all philosophy. In the Gita Krishna says: 'The unreal never is. The Real never is not. Men possessed of the knowledge of the Truth fully know these things.'

The meaning of Krishna's words is that a thing which never remains the same for any given period (such as the body) is unreal, and that the Real on the other hand always remains the same, fixed, immutable. All of the phenomenal world must therefore be unreal because everything in it is subject to change and decay. Only that which is unchanging is the Real and that is the divine spark within every human being or in other words the Soul or Self. This in the Gita is known as the Atman.

The Gita explains the six kinds of modifications to which matter is subject: birth, subsistence, growth, transformation, decay, and death. Of the Atman, or Soul or Self, Krishna says,

This Self weapons cut not; this Atman fire burns not; This water drowns not; and This wind dries not.

This Self is changeless, all-pervading, unmoving, immovable, the Atman is eternal. This Self is infinite and partless, so can be neither the subject nor the object of any action.

Some look upon the Atman and have understood it in all its wonder. Others can only speak of it though it is beyond their comprehension. Still others know of the Atman only by hearsay, and there are still others who are told about it and do not understand.

The Atman is difficult to comprehend, so that those who see, hear and speak of it are small in number. The Atman cannot be manifested to any of the bodily senses, nor considered intellectually. It is knowable in itself but incomprehensible to the unenlightened. Krishna speaks further of it thus:

All things are either perishable or imperishable, but there is another, called the Atman, the Highest Self, which, pervading the three worlds, sustains them.

The three worlds Krishna refers to are Bhuh, which is the Earth, Bhuvah, known as the Mid-Region, and Svah, the Eternal Place. The Atman is known in this world and in the Vedas as the supreme Reality. He who realizes the Atman becomes truly wise and the purpose of his life is fulfilled.

18. *Is it true that Yoga builds a perfect physique?*

This question refers specifically, of course, to Hatha Yoga which is concerned with postures (of which it is said there are three thousand!) and a system of breathing exercises known as pranayama. The science of Hatha Yoga was evolved because it was understood by the ancient sages of India that the perfection of the body—its health, vitality, and beauty—depends upon a harmony of material elements. From this knowledge arose the principle that this harmony, when lost, can be restored by the achievement of a balance or proportion dislocated by disease, physical, mental or emotional disturbance.

Incidentally this theory was also evolved and elaborated upon by Aristotle a thousand years later, and from his time onwards the theory and practice of Greek medicine were largely governed by the same precepts.

Hatha Yoga is not a system which is designed to promote abnormal strength of limb or hardness of muscle. That comes within the scope of gymnastics and athletics. In Hatha Yoga there is no violence of movement whatsoever, the accent rather is on *control*, including the control of the breath, and perfect physical balance. The control of the breath (pranayama) is closely connected with the treatment of nervous tension and other emotional disorders, as well as diseases of the respiratory tract. The control of the body, the promotion of spinal flexibility, the principles of balance and moderation imparted by the Yoga teacher, these elements by their very nature tend to result in a mind and body in which all the systems essential to good health function normally. In such circumstances the body would tend towards perfection because of this perfect harmony of material elements, and this harmony is reflected in the poise of the head, the serenity of expression, and the aspect of general well-being which emanates from the Yoga adept. The individual has a feeling of being at peace with himself.

However, the grace and poise which seem to radiate from the Hatha Yoga adept, is, I am bound to say, merely a *bonus*. The system was designed for a purpose very different from the mere perfecting of the physical body, as I have already explained. There is no doubt, nevertheless, that the constant practice of Hatha Yoga does result in a physique of perfect health and proportion and as such can definitely be recommended for people who are only interested in improving their looks, both bodily and facial.

19. *Does the practice of Yoga make one any happier?*

This is another question which I am constantly asked, and the answer, I am glad to say, is definitely yes. The whole philosophy of Yoga is concerned not only with a passion for the inner meanings which underlie appearances, but also with a deep interest in human happiness and welfare. Yoga proclaims the unity of all existence, promotes greater peace of mind and well-being, and offers a way of life free from tension, strife, ignorance and fallacy.

It teaches a personal morality leading to purity, strength and gentleness of character, and a social ethic concerned with the good of all beings and with social stability and integration. It teaches that true morality begins with the development of awareness of the moral law within, of which Kant speaks, a point in human evolution which transforms the merely half-civilized man into a cultured and considerate citizen and member of the society in which he moves.

Freed from the thraldom of purely animal impulses, guided by logic and detached reasoning, accepting with cheerfulness and equanimity the responsibilities of social existence and enjoying the manifold pleasures which this brings about, Man can be the finest product of social evolution. This is his privilege, and his alone.

Yoga's aim is to lead the individual, irrespective of credal, social, racial or political affiliations, step by step to the realization of the highest and best in life. It teaches that this can be attained here and now, in this life, and that the wish for, and the ability to attain, the fullest possible expression of his highest Self is inherent in the nature of every human being.

30

20. *What is Mantra Yoga?*

This is the Hindu science of Vibration which influences the subconscious mind and affects our nervous reaction to people and things. Man has a natural love for, and affinity with, rhythm and Mantra Yoga was devised as a 'safety valve' for Man, who lives his life under pressure and who therefore needs some form of nervous release. It is a fact that, in centuries other than the present one, Man has lived his life under some form of pressure, mainly mental or emotional, and that since the time when Man was a savage, Mantra Yoga (or something corresponding to it) has been necessary to his well-being.

The brain of Man receives vibrations to which, after a time, his thought-waves respond. This is the Yoga theory of the Mantra, that a slow, soothing repetitive rhythm calms the mind and produces serenity. To practise Mantra Yoga it says in the Gita:

> OM, Tat, Sat: this has been declared to be the triple designation of Brahman by whom, it is said, were created in ancient India the seers, the Vedas and the sacrificial rites.

'OM' is always uttered, as directed by the scriptures, before the undertaking of any act of sacrifice, the giving of alms or the practice of any austerity such as fasting. 'OM' in this context always signifies willingness, as well as being the principal name of Brahman or the Supreme Self.

'Tat' means 'That', the Indefinable or the Absolute, that which can be described only indirectly. It is uttered by those seeking Liberation but who desire no reward for their actions—in other words, those who practise Karma Yoga. Like the sacred syllable, 'OM', it is uttered before the making of any form of sacrifice, the giving of alms, or the practice of some form of austerity.

'Sat' signifies Reality, perseverance, and that which is ever permanent. All actions dedicated to Brahman, like OM and Tat, are Sat.

It is explained in the Gita that if a man performs his acts of sacrifice or almsgiving, or practises any austerity, without directing his mind and faith towards Brahman by uttering the three syllables, 'OM, Tat, Sat', then his actions are what is known as 'asat' or unreal, and cannot produce any good result.

Krishna explains further to Arjuna:

Therefore, uttering 'OM' are the sacrifices, gifts and austerities as enjoined in the scriptures always begun by those who follow the Vedas.

Uttering 'Tat', without aiming at fruits, are the various acts of Yajna (austerity and almsgiving) performed by the seekers of Moksha (Liberation).

The word 'Sat' is used in the sense of reality and goodness, and so also, O Arjuna, is the word 'Sat' used in the sense of a gracious act.

Steadiness in Yajna is also called 'Sat', as also action in connection with these is called 'Sat'.

Thus, according to the laws of vibration, the mantra 'OM, Tat, Sat' repeated slowly and rhythmically has a soothing effect on the mind and induces serenity when the mind is in a state of agitation.

21. *What is the meaning of Brahman?*

According to the Indian scriptures, Brahman is the Absolute, the Supreme Truth of non-dualistic Vedanta. The Gita describes it as:

This, the Indweller, of the bodies of all, is ever indestructible.

22. *What is a Brahmin?*

This is a member of the priestly caste, the very highest caste in Hindu society. The four Hindu castes are the Brahmins, the Kshattriyas (warriors), the Vaishyas (merchants) and the Sudras (the servants). In the Gita these caste names are used with a more subtle and psychological significance:

The prophets and defenders, providers and servers.

Each caste, according to the Gita, has its own particular duties to perform for the good of society in general. Thus, Krishna says:

Serenity, self-control, austerity, purity, forbearance and also uprightness, knowledge, realization and faith are the duties of a Brahmin born of his nature.

Heroism, boldness, firmness, dexterity, bravery, generosity and lordliness are the duties of a warrior born of his nature.

Agriculture, cattle-rearing and trade are the duties of a merchant born of his nature.

Work of the nature of service is the duty of a Sudra born of his nature.

Devoted to his own duty a man attains perfection.

I must mention here that the Gita refers to women as being of a lower caste than the Brahmins.

23. *What is the meaning of the word prana?*

This is the vital breath which sustains life in a physical body, hence pranayama meaning the control of the breath. But prana also means the primal energy or force, of which the other physical forces are manifestations. In the ancient books of Yoga, prana is described as having five modifications, according to its five separate functions. These are as follows:

1. Prana, the vital energy that controls the breath.
2. Apana, the vital energy that digests food and drink.
3. Samana, the vital energy that carries nutrition all over the body.
4. Vyana, the vital energy that pervades the entire organism.
5. Udana, the vital energy that cleanses the stomach.

The existence of prana, or life-force, was known not only to the Vedic sages of India, but also to the ancient Hebrews, Tibetans, the Chinese, Japanese and Egyptians, and of course to the Greeks! Even the very earliest Christians were aware of a cosmic energy which they called by different names.

In the Book of Genesis the Hebrews called it 'neshemet ruach hayim' which means the breath and spirit of life. To this very day the Hebrew toast before drinking is 'lehayim' which means 'to life'.

24. *Is there any relationship between the type of food one eats and one's mental and physical state?*

You would get different answers to this question from a doctor, a dietician, a health-food devotee, or a person who has little interest in what he eats one way or another. So I will quote the Gita in answer to this one.

Krishna to Arjuna:

The foods which promote vitality, energy, strength, health, cheerfulness and appetite are those which are oily and savoury, and are liked by the Sattvika (those who are righteous).

The foods that are bitter, sour, saline, excessively hot, dry, pungent and burning produce pain, grief and disease and are liked by the Rajasika (restless and passionate men).

That which is stale, tasteless, putrid and impure is liked only by the Tamasika (men who are dull and slothful).

According to the Gita, food is 'stale' if cooked more than three hours beforehand. That is 'putrid' which is left on the plate after a meal. Food that is cooked overnight is also regarded as inferior.

25. *Is it true to say that Truth is Absolute, but that the Concept of Truth varies with the individual consciousness?*

No one can say when the ultimate Truth has been reached because it is impossible to determine when the individual consciousness has been developed to a point where further development is impossible. So according to Yoga, Truth itself is absolute but the concept of it does vary with the individual consciousness. But I would point out here that truth is not a matter of belief but of demonstration. Neither is it a question of authority but of perception.

26. *Is the 'Bad' in Philosophy merely an imaginary manifestation of thought or could it be described as wrong but in fact real?*

The 'bad' in philosophy is by no means an imaginary entity, it is more proper to describe it as a perversion. To use an analogy, electricity is neither bad nor good. Used for light or for power to drive engines we call it 'good'. If we grasp an improperly insulated wire and receive a shock it simply means that we were either careless or *ignorant* of the basic laws which govern electricity.

In the same way, the one Infinite Power, which in Yoga is known as the source of all Power, is manifest in our lives, and it is displayed as either good or bad according to whether we make use of it constructively or destructively.

27. *If the real 'Self' as described in the Bhagavad Gita is a spiritual fact and therefore perfect, and since it controls and directs both mind and body, why is Man such an imperfect creature?*

This is a question I am asked very often as so many people are perplexed by the world as we now find it with all its war and tension and worry. The answer ties in with the answer to the previous question.

Spiritual Law always operates as perfectly as mathematics, that is with immutable precision. If the individual thinks constructively, then the results will also be constructive and harmonious. If, on the other hand, he thinks destructively, he reaps exactly what he sows. The Spiritual Law itself works precisely, and what we see are not imperfect results. We are free to *choose* what we think, but the resulting thoughts are governed by a Law which is unchangeable.

A quotation from an Ode by Sadi (1193–1291) will illustrate this point.

We have planted thorns; shall we gather dates? We have spun coarse wool: shall we weave fine brocade therefrom? . . .

Our passions are our own destruction. And O, the bewailing on the Day of resurrection!
Our life so precious is past and cannot return; and we still are in sin!
How weak and unmanly to sink and settle in this world whereon brave men only travel; but make it not their home . . .

Perchance from the store-house of the grain of grace of the Saints a single ear of corn will be given to us as a gift:
We have not sown it ourselves.

Translated by JUAN MASCARÓ

28. *Why do Yoga pupils have to stand on their heads?*

This is a fallacy. They do not *have* to stand on their heads. One can practise Yoga successfully without performing this famous posture, in fact I prefer my own pupils not to do it unless I am standing beside them to correct any faults, because such an unnatural posture *can* be dangerous—you can fall and hurt yourself, you can strain your neck or your back—and the very thought of standing on their heads makes some people intensely nervous. For all these reasons I never insist on my own pupils performing the headstand. If, on the other hand, they specifically request that I demonstrate it in order that they might perform it themselves, then of course I will do so. I discuss it at length on pages 74–80 of my book *Yoga and Your Health* and demonstrate it in photographs 26–29.

But *why* do Yoga pupils stand on their heads if this is not Man's natural position? First of all it affects the four most important endocrine glands in the body—the pituitary, the pineal, the thyroid and the parathyroid, those glands which keep the entire body mechanism in perfect order. It is said to be a relaxing exercise and yet many people who perform it point out, and with justification, that at first it is anything but relaxing. It causes tension in the neck and a feeling of general unease.

So let me first point out the beneficial results of performing the headstand. The direct result of the various dangers which threaten the general well-being of our physical and mental mechanism is stress. The most powerful, and therefore the most dangerous of these stress factors are our own emotions. Recent physical and psychological research has thrown new light on the function of the pituitary gland in particular and its ability to activate the body's defences against any kind of alien influence; stress can, without doubt, be described as the most insidious of these influences.

How does the headstand combat these influences? First of all it requires some practice to perform it if you cannot already do it. And the repeated forward bending and straightening of the legs and spine of the first two stages, combined with deep and rhythmical breathing, strengthens the spine, lungs and neck and reorientates the circulation of the blood. The achievement of the full headstand, after the right kind of supervision and practice, results in a surge of self-confidence which is very beneficial psychologically. Stress, and the resulting fits of depression and ill temper, are very damaging to the nervous system as a whole and therefore to the entire mechanism of the body, so that anything which helps to combat this is beneficial.

The inversion of the body results in an increased supply of blood to the brain and every vital organ of the head, including the pituitary gland. It therefore increases mental and physical efficiency, and as a bonus, the digestive function is also improved.

But to reiterate the warning I made in *Yoga and Your Health*, the headstand should not, *at any time*, be attempted by people with any kind of heart trouble, ear infections, especially chronic infections of the ears, high or low blood pressure, catarrh or sinus trouble or any form of eye trouble. It can do more harm than good and in fact can be extremely dangerous.

For those who, in spite of everything I have said, insist on practising the headstand because they feel they will benefit from it, I would suggest that the position should not be held for too long at a time. The best way to obtain beneficial results would be to execute a series of headstands, smoothly and rhythmically, each to a count of ten, or to be more precise, for exactly ten seconds. In this way, the headstand can be performed up to twenty times, but the student should stop as soon as he feels tired. The body should not be made to perform strenuous exercises when it is ready to take a rest. This is a rule of Hatha Yoga which does not apply to any other form of physical culture.

Ideally, the headstand should be performed in conjunction with slow and rhythmical deep breathing, but this technique is best imparted personally by a Yoga teacher, who would be likely to have taught his pupil some of the pranayama exercises, before attempting to teach the headstand. I repeat, it is by far the wisest policy not to attempt this exercise without expert instruction.

29. *It is said that almost anyone can benefit from the practice of Yoga. Why then is one of the chapters in the Bhagavad Gita called, 'Kingly Knowledge and Kingly Secret'?*

The chapter in the Gita with the above heading is the ninth, but as early as the fourth chapter, Krishna says to Arjuna:

I have this day told thee this same ancient Yoga for thou art
My devotee and also My friend, and this secret is profound

indeed.

The interpretation of the word 'secret' in this context is that the profound knowledge of Yoga is not the privilege of any one individual or sect—it is secret because of its very profundity. People, as it were, get the Yoga they deserve, that is they reap exactly what they sow, and people who have not the intellect, the patience, or the necessary faith to discover exactly how profound this Yoga is dismiss it as some esoteric secret available to a privileged few. But this is in no way true. It is 'secret' only to those who are unworthy —that is those who lack perseverance.

The ninth chapter begins with Krishna saying to Arjuna:

> To thee, who dost not reject, verily shall I now teach thee this most secret knowledge, united with realization, knowing which thou shalt be free from ignorance forever.

And further on Krishna says:

> Unaware of My higher state, as the great Lord of beings, *only fools* deride and disregard me in my human form.

I would remind my readers here that Krishna is the God Vishnu who appears to Arjuna in his human form, that Arjuna may see Him the more easily and not be completely dazzled.

Krishna continues:

> Those of vain hopes and efforts, of vain knowledge, and without logic, they verily are deluded.

The meaning of this sentence is as follows:

'Of vain hopes'—those who entertain futile hopes that there is a God other than myself who would bestow favours more quickly turn away from Me and their efforts are therefore of no avail. Likewise, the efforts of these people, because of their turning away, are ineffectual.

'Of vain knowledge'—those people whose knowledge of the scriptures is based on fallacious reasoning are, in fact, ignorant.

'Without logic' speaks for itself. People who have not the gift of logic or who have not taken the trouble to cultivate it are the ones who are easily deluded and whose discrimination between

38

the Real and the unreal is clouded.

Krishna continues thus:

> Those who know the Vedas, purified from sins by drinking the
> Soma juice, worshipping Me with sacrifices, they reach the
> world of the Lord of the Devas.

'Soma juice': this plant (perhaps an asclepiad) has an intoxicating
juice which was used in ancient Indian religious ceremonies, and
was considered to be a manifestation of God.

'Lord of the Devas': Devas, literally 'shining ones', are the gods
of Hindu mythology. Indra is the King of these gods and is also
known as Shatakratu because he had performed one hundred
sacrifices.

Krishna says in the next verse:

> Thus, abiding by the injunctions of the Vedas . . . to them thus
> ever zealously engaged, I carry what they lack and preserve
> what they already have.

'Abiding by the injunctions of the Vedas' means performing the
rituals and the Karmakanda (the part of the Vedas which is concerned with rituals and sacrifices).

'I carry what they lack and preserve what they already have'
means that Krishna secures gain and safety for such people.

The above answer will, I hope, demonstrate to my readers, how
every single word in the Bhagavad Gita requires study and interpretation and understanding, and this applies also to the Vedas
and the Upanishads. It therefore follows that a person who cannot
apply himself to such hard study and concentration would naturally regard Yoga as 'secret'. Its inner meaning would be hidden
from him, but Yoga is in fact no secret to those who have the
patience to study it properly.

30. *Will I ever be able to learn Hatha Yoga if I cannot sit in the
     Lotus Posture?*

Some people have a positive fixation about Yoga's two best-known
postures, the Lotus and the headstand. They are, in fact, two of
the more difficult postures, and with regard to the Lotus, to anyone

over the age of about eighteen years, it is extremely painful and formidable, though adepts make it look so easy. It is not easy to anyone who has not been used to sitting that way since childhood, unless they are what is known as 'double-jointed', or unless they have kept the hip-joints flexible through some form of athletics, gymnastics, or ballet.

Anyone beginning the study of Hatha Yoga who cannot sit in the Lotus posture is extremely unlikely ever to be able to do so. Even the Half-Lotus would present difficulties. But I repeat, this would not normally apply to anyone under the age of about eighteen, though I have known one or two people of only sixteen who could not bend their legs sufficiently to be able to sit even in the Easy Pose, that is with the feet tucked under the legs in tailor fashion.

But it is perfectly possible to become an adept at Hatha Yoga even though the hip-joints are so seized up that the Lotus posture is impossible to achieve. Yoga teachers know how to circumvent this difficulty though it is always a hard task to convince the disappointed pupil of this!

31. *Will you explain exactly what the Vedas and the Upanishads are?*

The Vedas are the most sacred scriptures of the Hindus and the ultimate authority of the Hindu religion and philosophy. They are reputed to have been arranged in their present form by Vyasa, a celebrated sage who is also believed to be the author of the eighteen Puranas (the Books of Hindu Mythology); the Brahma-sutras (an authoritative treatise on Vedanta philosophy) and the Mahabharata (the Hindu epic in which is embodied the Bhagavad Gita).

I am frankly sceptical about this last because the Mahabharata is reputed to be the longest poem in the world: in its original form it was said to be twenty-four thousand verses in length and it grew to something like one hundred thousand verses. It is, like the Old Testament, a collection of narratives and it is unlikely to be a homogeneous work. But it is *possible* that Vyasa is the author of the Bhagavad Gita.

In the Vedas we see the dawn of spiritual insight. They were arranged into four books, the Rig-Veda, the Yajur-Veda, the Sama-Veda and the Atharva-Veda.

In the Upanishads we see a progression from the dawn of spiritual insight to the fullest splendour of inner vision. The Upanishads form one of the sections of the Vedas and contain the basic philosophy of the Vedanta (see Question 5 of this chapter). There are said to be one hundred and eight Upanishads of which eleven are the most important. The eleven are: the Aitareya, the Taittiriya, the Chanddogya, the Brihadaranyaka, the Mundaka, the Mandukya, the Isa, the Kena, the Katha, the Prasna, and the Svetasvatara.

The word Upanishad is generally thought to mean commentary but it is derived from a Sanskrit word meaning 'gathered around'. In ancient days, when there were no written records and philosophy was imparted from teacher to pupils by word of mouth, the pupils gathered round their teacher to hear his discourses. Those Upanishads which have come down to us are condensed records of these discourses, and they are often brief and cryptic in form to such an extent that a vast literature has grown up about them.

However, the Vedas, in their original form, are even more cryptic than the Upanishads so that the latter are considered the more valuable books of Vedic literature. As I have mentioned, the Upanishads contain the basic philosophy of the Vedanta, though the philosophy was later developed by such thinkers as Vyasa, Gaudapada (whose principal work is a commentary on the Mandukya Upanishad), S'ankara, Ramanuja and Madhva (who we know lived from 1199–1276 A.D.). Ramanuja himself wrote no commentaries on the Upanishads though several of his pupils have done so.

It is interesting to observe that the ancient seers of the Vedas included both men and women, lay people and sannyasins (Hindu monks), and people outside the Brahmin caste. Many revisions of the Vedas have been lost to us and those Vedic teachers who are at present known to us were mostly lay people or householders. There is no agreement among Hindu or Western scholars regarding the date of the Vedas.

The ancient Hindus divided the lifetime of the individual into four stages. The first one was known as brahmacarya, the period of study, during which time the young man lived with his teacher, practised various disciplines and austerities, and closely observed nature. He was also expected to commit to memory the texts of the Vedas!

The second stage was known as garhasthya, the life of the householder. As a husband and citizen he performed his civic duties according to his position in the Hindu caste system.

The third stage was known as vanaprastha, the life of the forest-dweller, though he was still, technically, a householder and as such had to perform certain daily sacrifices obligatory for all but the sannyasins. This was a stage of symbolic worship enjoined in the Vedas, and profound meditation.

The fourth and last stage was known as sannyasa, the monastic life, when the individual gave up the world wholly in search of Truth. Sannyasins were outside all castes and beyond all social conventions. They became, ultimately, spiritual teachers, their lives dedicated to service of their fellow men. These men were obliged to study the Upanishads constantly, and this monastic life was considered to be the natural culmination of the three preceding stages.

32. *What are the so-called Four Qualifications of the Yoga Pupil?*

Vedantic teachers insist that genuine seekers after Knowledge, the really serious students of Yoga, must practise proper disciplines of which there are four. They are:

1. Viveka (discrimination between the Real and the unreal). Without this discipline the following one is impossible.

2. Vairagya (renunciation). This entails the absolute disregard of all pleasures, earthly and otherwise. The reason for this discipline is that all pleasures are the results of finite action, and this includes even benign action such as charity, study and worship. The explanation of this severe discipline is that the Vedanta seeks to remove ignorance, the one barrier to the highest Knowledge or the realization of the immutable Self, which is in no way the result of any kind of action.

3. Satsampatti (the six treasures), which form the ethical basis of the spiritual life. The practice of this discipline prepares the innate faculties of the mind for the reception of higher knowledge. They are as follows:

(a) Sama (calmness). This means that the pupil should detach his mind from all objects perceived by the senses through the understanding of their inherent defects. Having achieved this detachment the pupil then either studies the scriptures or listens to his guru (teacher) instructing him about them. He must then reason out the meaning of the scriptures for himself and having done so should meditate upon this meaning.

(b) Dama (self-control). This entails the restraint of all organs of perception and action, the detachment of them from their respective objects, and the keeping of them under strict control. This frees the mind for meditation and reason.

(c) Uparati (translated as 'self-settledness'). This requires the pupil to relinquish all wordly duties and to accept the monastic life.

(d) Titiksa (forbearance). This is the endurance of all physical and mental afflictions.

The above four disciplines are referred to by Krishna in the Gita as follows:

When the completely controlled mind rests serenely in the Self alone, free from longing after all things, then one is called stead-fast in the Self.

When the mind, absolutely restrained by the practice of concentration, and when seeing the Self by the self is satisfied in his own Self; when he feels that infinite bliss, perceived by the purified intellect and which transcends the senses, and established wherein he never departs from his real state; and having obtained which, regards no other acquisition to that, and where established, he is not moved even by heavy sorrow—let that be known as the state called by the name of Yoga—a state of severance from the contact of pain. This Yoga should be practised with perseverence, undisturbed by depression of heart.

The remaining two of the six treasures to which I have referred are as follows:

(e) Samadhana (complete concentration). This is achieved only after (a) to (d) have been mastered to the teacher's satisfaction.

(f) Sraddha (faith). The pupil must be in a mental state to accept fully the words of the Vedanta. This faith or belief is not blind and unquestioning, it is a positive attitude of mind, where the pupil knows that he is fully capable of making any sacrifice for his belief.

4. The last of the four qualifications of the Yoga pupil, according to the Vedantic teachers, is Mumuksutvam or the longing for Liberation. This means that the pupil longs to free himself from the bondage of his bodily self, from the will and from the ego both

of which cloud his judgement. This longing for Liberation is the
result of the preceding disciplines outlined above.

33. *What does Self-Control in Yoga involve?*

Self-control forms the very kernel of Vedantic discipline, and
without it no spiritual progress is possible. It means the emptying
of the mind of all worldly things and then, through contemplation,
filling up the resulting vacuum with the spirit of Brahman or
Truth.

I should emphasize that self-control should, in every way, be
distinguished from the practice of meaningless penances and austerities. Above all self-torture is condemned. The Gita says:

> Those men who practise severe austerities not enjoined by the
> Shastras, given to ostentation and egoism, senselessly torture all
> the organs in the body, and Me dwelling as I do in the body
> within, these men outrage me by their demonic nature.

The real nature of self-control is the strengthening of the faculties
of discrimination, will-power, and determination. What is enjoined with great emphasis is *not* the weakening of the body and
the mind through self-chastisement. In parts of India especially it
is possible to come across street performers, daring to call themselves Yogis, who perform revolting acts of self-torture such as
walking on spikes or burning coals, sticking knives into themselves,
drinking acid, and letting their arms wither in the sun and wind.
These people are nothing more than circus performers except that
such spectacles are hardly suitable for children and are no more
entertaining to adults. It is distressing to any serious student of
Yoga that such distorted ideas are prevalent in India, and sincere
Yoga devotees do their utmost to discourage such misleading and
dangerous exhibitions.

The uninformed think that Yoga is merely a system of physical
exercises and, particularly in the West, no form of Yoga is more
popular (or more misunderstood) than Hatha Yoga, the physical
discipline. Its popularity is quite understandable because of its
basic principle of the health of the body, but I must stress that Hatha
Yoga is only an adjunct (although an important one) to all the
other systems of Yoga. The physical body is the only instrument we

have and is the vessel of the mind, so it is only common sense to keep it as free from disease and pain as possible.

No Yoga teacher expects his pupils to perform feats of endurance or contort his limbs so as to cause unnecessary distress. The system is always adapted to suit the age, needs, and capabilities of the individual and at no time, as in ballet, gymnastics and other forms of physical culture, is any violence of movement involved. Hatha Yoga, as is the case with all forms of Yoga, goes *with* the body and not against it. Economy of energy is practised at all times as any adept of Hatha Yoga can demonstrate. This is as much a part of the self-control of Yoga as is the disciplining of the mind.

There are three lines by Tennyson which aptly express the Yogic principle of self-control:

> Self-reverence, self-knowledge, self-control,
> These three alone lead life to sovereign power
> . . . .
> Acting the law we live by without fear.

Two lines by Robert Burns express it even more succinctly:

> Prudent, cautious self-control
> Is wisdom's root.

34. *There are said to be Four Ideals in Yoga by which Man can make his life more pleasant in this day and age. Will you explain what these are?*

The four ideals of Yoga which serve the ends of human endeavour are known as dharma, artha, kama, and moksa. In Western and modern parlance these may be described as follows.

Dharma means righteousness and should be the basis of all Man's actions. If it is so, then it is in harmony with the innate temperament of the individual whatever this may be, as Man's nature, according to Yoga, contains a divine spark. Therefore, if a person thinks and acts righteously at all times he will naturally evolve spiritually and will attain success in all he undertakes.

Artha means wealth, and it may surprise some readers that this is not frowned upon by the Vedic sages. On the contrary, wealth is regarded not only as an effective means of self-expression in life, and in one's inter-personal relationships, but as a perfectly reasonable goal of pursuit at some stage of a man's life. But it is strictly enjoined by the Vedic sages that wealth must be acquired only by dharma or righteousness otherwise it will serve no spiritual purpose and will, in fact lead to greed and a striving after power. The Gita is quite specific about this point. Krishna speaks as follows:

> Forsaking egoism, power, pride, lust and property, freed from the notion of 'mine'; and tranquil—he alone is fit to become Brahman.

Kama is the fulfilment of both aesthetic and sensuous aspirations. This too must be guided by righteousness lest it degenerate into hedonism.

While the disciplines of Yoga do not require a man to forgo dharma, artha, and kama, which is where Yoga is an innately humane and realistic philosophy applicable to any day and age, it does issue a warning that the satisfaction derived from worldly success, the achievement of wealth, and the enjoyment of beauty is in no way enduring and ultimately cannot satisfy Man's inner need. This can only be fulfilled by the fourth of Yoga's ideals, namely moksa, which means Liberation.

The first three of the Ideals belong essentially to the material world, but the fourth belongs to that region above that which is merely material and therefore ephemeral, namely the realm of the Soul, Spirit or Self. Therefore the fourth Ideal is the crowning achievement of human life. Here is what Krishna in the Gita has to say about it:

> Relinquishing all dharmas take refuge in Me alone; I will liberate thee, Arjuna. Leave behind thee all worldly things and dedicate thy life to Me, for I alone can give thee liberty from the bonds of all thy past actions. Thou hast cause to rejoice.

35. *It seems however much one studies Yoga and philosophises about Man's Higher Self, in actual everyday life we suffer—when we are ill, when loved ones are ill or die, at angry words, at disappointments. Is this not so?*

From time immemorial Man has been struggling to eliminate

suffering from life on this earth. How far he has been successful we can see from the wars and misery all around us. The average person, with all his human weaknesses, finds his actions almost always at variance with his ideals and aspirations. This is because what Yoga says is true—Man does have a higher Self, but it can only be realized by controlling and transcending his lower or earthly self. This requires a great deal of hard work.

Despite the neuroticizing tendencies of modern life, all is not lost. Life is always a challenge, and we do have a choice as to how we conduct our lives. One way leads towards the ideal: the brotherhood of man, which has been the aim of every religious and philosophical movement the world has ever seen. The other way leads in exactly the opposite direction. Man does not have to be a human turnip, or sit and bewail his lot. He can make a conscious choice. He suffers because he is not aware that he *has* this choice.

Yoga does not claim, and never has claimed, to have the monopoly on how to live a good life, but it certainly is more practical and straightforward than some other systems whose aims are almost identical with those of Yoga. Basically Yoga accepts the life situation as we find it and suggests methods by which we can transcend our human limitations.

36. *What is Kriya Yoga?*

It is closely linked to meditation and is very popular in India. It is hardly known about in the West, and as well as being closely linked to meditation it is, in actual fact, a form of Bhakti Yoga. It appeals to people to whom nothing matters except the steady, daily advancement of the spiritual side of their nature, and is considered in India to be a powerful instrument through which human evolution can be quickened.

The sages of ancient India discovered that one of the secrets of heightened consciousness is linked with the control of the breath, which is called pranayama. So Kriya Yoga basically involves three disciplines: meditation, the inner repetition of the sound OM, and the freeing of the life-force, which is ordinarily absorbed in maintaining the beating of the heart, for higher activities by a singular method of stilling the ceaseless demands of the breath. This last discipline can be dangerous unless practised under the expert eye of a Guru because its methods, although aiming at spiritual advancement, are nevertheless highly technical.

I have included this question on Kriya Yoga because of the number of times I have been asked about it, but I certainly would strongly advise anyone in the West against attempting to practise this form of Yoga.

37. *It is said that there are Five Daily Duties enjoined on Hindu Householders. What are these?*

1. Deva-Yajna, which means offering sacrifices to the gods.

2. Brahma-Yajna, which means reciting the scriptures and teaching them to others.

3. Pitri-Yajna, which means the offering of libations of water to one's ancestors.

4. Nri-Yajna, which is the feeding of those who need food.

5. Bhuta-Yajna, which means the feeding of the lower animals.

These are the five duties of householders according to the Bhagavad Gita. The performance of them is said to free householders from the five inevitable sins connected with the killing of life by using the following five household utensils—the water-jar, the mortar and pestle, the oven, the broom and the grinding-stone.

38. *Does Yoga help to build character?*

Yes, it helps to iron out the deficiencies in a person's character, strengthen weaknesses, and tones down the more aggressive traits. In other words it 'evens things up'.

Let us take a hypothetical 'ideal' man. What would be the dominant factors which make up his personality? Common sense and courage would be high on the list, so would honesty, a sense of humour, and a well-developed sense of social duty. Add to this modesty, tolerance, generosity, patience, self-control and sympathy and we have someone more like an angel than a human being! However, there are some of the characteristics of our hypothetical man.

What of the other side of the coin? What is he not? To begin with, he is not so engrossed in his work that he cannot find the time to widen his horizons. He is not so fond of wealth as to make it the goal of his life. His interest in people is not confined to the narrow circle of his family. He is neither rude nor aggressive towards others, but neither is he over-sentimental.

A glance at the above will show us how far our own characters deviate from the ideal. Yet most people would like to be nearer to it than they are. So how would Yoga's methods deal with a situation of this kind?

There are several stages through which the pupil can be trained to eradicate undesirable character traits and build up the weak ones. Let us take an example of the former.

1. By close observance of his own character, the student would gradually become aware of his worst defect or what he considers it to be. He must fully accept the situation, however unpleasant, and however much it injures his own self-esteem.

2. By constant observance and training the defective faculty can not only be eradicated but can become, in time, a superior and dominant character trait. For example, if you discover that your worst character trait is intolerance, the conscious and constant practice of tolerance would become, in time, second nature.

3. The pupil would then be required to place himself deliberately in situations where he would either have to exercise tolerance or show up his excessive intolerance to everyone in sight. Naturally he would tend to take the former course, not wishing to lose his friends or to 'lose face'. At this stage the pupil's ego is still very much to the fore.

4. Having trained himself over a considerable period of time to exercise tolerance on every possible occasion until it becomes second nature, the pupil would then be instructed by his teacher to translate his newly acquired desirable character trait into some form of socially useful behaviour. What form this would take would be the choice of the pupil himself—there is much useful work to be done in the world.

5. Having rid himself of an undesirable character trait, the pupil then has to start all over again, discover another, and go through the whole process again. And so on, until all defects in his character have been translated into socially useful behaviour.

Perhaps more intimidating is the building up of weak character traits, but the same method applies. Either way it is a laborious process and requires much patience.

39. *In the Aphorisms of Patanjali it is said that Eight Disciplines are enunciated as necessary to the achievement of Self-Awareness. What are these?*

1. Yama (general self-discipline) which encompasses non-violence, non-injury, non-stealing, purity, and the non-acceptance of gifts.

The meaning of non-injury is that neither by thought, word nor deed shall the student of Yoga do harm to any person or other living thing so far as possible. The acceptance of gifts can create obligations which can be disturbing to the awakening consciousness. The other disciplines speak for themselves.

2. Niyama (particular self-discipline) closely resembles the three Sabbath practises of Judaism: rest, holiness, and joy. Patanjali also advocates cleanliness, austerity and meditation.

3. Asana (posture). This is the best-known form of Yoga discipline in the Western world. It calls for stringent physical discipline and is conducive to physical and mental relaxation, health of body and peace of mind.

4. Pranayama (the control of the breath). This includes slow, deep breathing, inwards and outwards, and the retention of the breath. Pranayama stills the mind but on no account should it be practised unless under the expert tuition of a Yoga teacher.

5. Pratyahara (self-withdrawal). This is the detachment of the senses from material things.

6. Dharana, which means concentration.

7. Dhyana, which is meditation. I have discussed this in detail in a later chapter.

8. Samadhi—this is the highest stage of Yoga, an ecstatic, trance-like state, involving complete concentration. It is a state of transcendent consciousness which is said to bring complete enlightenment.

Chapter 2

THE YOGA OF THE BHAGAVAD GITA

Behold, I find You
Where the ploughman breaks through the hard soil,
Where the quarryman explodes stone out of the hillside,
Where the miner digs metals out of the reluctant earth,
Where men earn their bread by the sweat of their brow,
Among the lonely and the poor, the lowly, the lost,
You are with them in blazing heat and shattering storm.

Behold, I find You
In the mind free to sail by its own star,
In words that spring from the depth of truth,
Where endeavour reaches undespairing for perfection,
Wherever men struggle for justice and freedom,
Where the scientist toils to unravel the secrets of Your world,
Where the poet makes beauty out of words,
Wherever noble deeds are done.

RABINDRANATH TAGORE *Gitanjali*
Translated by Rabbi Chaim Stern from
David Frischmann's Hebrew version

THE BHAGAVAD GITA has an undisputed place among the world's greatest literature. Written originally in Sanskrit, and the first work to be translated from Sanskrit into English, it is a religio-philosophical poem in eighteen chapters. The title means, 'The Song of the Blessed One' or 'The Song of God'.

The study of the Sanskrit language inevitably leads philologists to the discovery that Greek, Latin, the Germanic, Slavonic and the Celtic languages, together with Persian and Sanskrit itself can all be traced to a primitive and wholly unwritten language called Aryan. About 300 years B.C. the first complete Sanskrit grammar was written by a man named Panini.

Scholars soon became aware that Sanskrit literature contains works of the highest order, among them the great songs of the Vedas which were composed long before writing was introduced into India, the Upanishads, some of the principal canonical books of Hinduism, and the poetry and dramas of Kalidasa (circa 400 A.D.), one of the most illustrious figures in classic Sanskrit literature and one of the greatest of all Oriental poets. There is also the epic poem, the 'Mahabharata', reputed to be about twenty times as long as Milton's *Paradise Lost*! The Bhagavad Gita is incorporated into this vast work and forms the 25th to the 42nd chapters.

Sanskrit literature also contains the famous epic, the 'Ramayana', the work of Manu, the celebrated law-giver of ancient India who is generally supposed to have written the 'Code of Manu'.

There is also the scientific philosophy of the Sankhya, a great body of lyrical drama and poetry, the psychological philosophy of Yoga, the philosophy of the Vedanta, and many stories, parables and fables which are still told in India today.

Much of Sanskrit literature is enlaced with idealism, but also with an astonishingly practical wisdom which is as applicable to our own age as to the time when it was composed. Throughout this literature we find the typically Indian thirst for spiritual insight. Perhaps what fascinates scholars about Sanskrit literature is the fact that the collective mind of India, from ancient times, has never ceased in its search for Enlightenment.

But scholars of comparative religion have always found two vital points of contact between all the highest of the world's beliefs. One is that the goal and purpose of Man's life is the search for, and discovery of, Truth, and that this Truth can be experienced by direct but super-rational means. The second is that there have always been human incarnations of what may be called the God-head, and this has been stated over the centuries in a multitude of ways and languages. The Bhagavad Gita is such a statement, per-haps one of the most beautiful and unequivocal.

Psychologists, in fact all those who study human nature, have always been aware that people differ widely in temperament, ability, and intellectual and spiritual potential. Some people are quite obviously at a higher stage of spiritual evolution than others, and this fact is made quite clear in the Bhagavad Gita, especially in the section on the three gunas. (I refer my readers to Question 9 of the first chapter of this book.)

The subject matter of the Mahabharata is concerned with the

concepts of good and evil and is set against a background of war. But my concern here is not to dwell upon this vast epic (which would require a whole book in itself), but to make the episode in its sixth book—the Bhagavad Gita—more accessible to my readers, to indicate a way through its exotic phraseology to its essential and timeless humanity.

The main part of the Gita itself is a dialogue between a warrior Prince, Arjuna, and his chosen deity, the god Vishnu in his human form of Krishna. The name Krishna is derived from the word, 'krish' which means to scrape or to draw away. Krishna is so called because he draws away all imperfections from those who are devoted to him. The dialogue contains the essence of Self-Knowledge, and a detailed exploration of ethics, and examines the relationship in the human mind between appearance and reality.

The dialogue form itself was favoured by Plato and other great philosophical writers as a vivid and dramatic means of exploring every possible aspect of an intellectual argument which might otherwise become too abstruse and protracted. The Gita then is a dramatic poem and it has also been compared to a great symphony, so musical is its language and so dominant its concept of harmony. It has many themes: the attainment of freedom by the performance of one's duty in life; that Man has the faculty of reason to enable him to distinguish true emotion from mere emotionalism; self-control, self-knowledge, self-harmony, and above all the four Yogas, Raja, Jnana, Karma and Bhakti. And when we think that all this is contained in a book of no great length we begin to understand why the Gita has fascinated thinking people for well over two thousand years. Scholars differ as to the actual date of the writing of it and it may not now be possible to date it exactly, but one can, with impunity, say that it was written approximately five hundred years B.C.

The work is divided into three sections, each containing six chapters. The first section deals with the duties and observances of caste which are shown to be in accord with the principles of Yoga philosophy. The second section contains the pantheistic doctrine of the Vedanta, and in the third section these are interwoven with a description of the state of highest knowledge which is the aim of all Yoga.

From this broad outline we can now approach the Gita in more detail. A cursory glance at the book will reveal the extraordinary

53

beauty of its language. It has been translated hundreds of times, and some translations are more poetic than others, but the essential music of the Gita remains indestructible. This fact alone would set the work apart as a piece of great writing.

Some translations, especially those done by Indian scholars, begin with a meditation of which the first word is the basic sound OM which I discussed in the first chapter of this book.

> OM O Bhagavad Gita. O Loving Mother
> upon Thee I meditate.

And there follows a salutation to the Gita and to the god Krishna 'of mighty intellect and with eyes large like the petals of a full-blown lotus' and whose compassion 'makes eloquent the mute and the cripple cross mountains'.

One is reminded here of the words Handel set to music in his *Messiah*: 'Then shall the eyes of the blind be opened, and the ears of the deaf unstopped, and the tongues of the dumb shall sing.' Indeed there is a remarkable similarity between many of the concepts and expressions of the Gita and those of the Old and New Testaments.

After the salutation there is an invocation in which Krishna is called 'Guru of the Worlds', and in which we learn the names of some who fought in the great battle which forms part of the subject matter of the Mahabharata. Here begins the Gita proper and at once the situation is set out before us. The first pages continue in the same tone as the Mahabharata itself and so vivid is the language that we can almost hear the sound of trumpets and kettle-drums and cowhorns, the rattle of chariot wheels, the shouts of the warriors, and the snorting and neighing of the white horses yoked to the chariots. The noise is tremendous, and then we hear the sound of a conch-shell which signifies the beginning of the battle, and then the sound of many conches, and with all this clamour vibrating in our ears, Arjuna himself, full of the spirit of war, emerges to the forefront of the drama.

His first words are addressed to his charioteer:

Place my chariot, O Achyuta, between the two armies that I may see those who stand there prepared for war. In this preparation for battle let me know with whom I shall have to fight.

The name 'Achyuta' means the Changeless One, in other words Lord Krishna. It is fascinating to note that throughout the Gita, Arjuna's relationship with Krishna has a dual nature. On the one hand Krishna is Arjuna's charioteer whom he treats sometimes as a friend and equal; at other times he suddenly remembers Krishna's real nature and is appalled at his own presumption at treating his God as a fellow human-being.

So in the first instance we see Arjuna in fact requesting Krishna to do his bidding, and then suddenly with a shock he sees that those against whom he must fight are his own kinsmen. His attitude towards Krishna changes. He addresses his charioteer as Govinda, the One who gives Enlightenment, and so we know that Arjuna is well aware who Krishna really is. But we also learn that he sometimes forgets. For instance, in the second chapter, when Krishna urges Arjuna not to let his emotions cloud his judgement:

Yield not to unmanliness, Arjuna. Ill doth it become thee. Cast off thy faint-heartedness and arise.

Arjuna actually disobeys Krishna and says to him,

I will not fight.

And this after Arjuna has called upon Krishna for help with the words,

Say decidedly where my duty lies, O Krishna. I am Thy disciple. Instruct me who have taken refuge in Thee.

His declaration, 'I am Thy disciple' is important because until it is made the Master may not impart the highest knowledge. And so we find, right at the beginning of the instruction that Arjuna earnestly begs for, that he is human enough to disobey his own teacher!

It has surprised many of my pupils that the setting of the Gita is a battlefield, but as the layers of meaning are unfolded and understood, it becomes apparent to us that this battle is of a very different order from that depicted in the Mahabharata. The Gita describes a battle for an inner victory, the struggle of a human soul upwards, with the utmost difficulty, towards the highest knowledge and beyond that even—to the harmony with all things which we call Yoga, and through Yoga to Liberation.

Because of the tremendous inner struggle facing Arjuna, as would be the case for any mortal, it is hardly surprising that, in the beginning, Arjuna is sceptical of the words of his own teacher and, wallowing in his own misery and confusion, is inclined to be disobedient. Any Yoga teacher in this day and age would be able to recount instances of similar behaviour from pupils, anxious to learn Yoga but new to the subject. So too, throughout the Gita, we can find instances of this twofold attitude which Arjuna has towards Krishna until, in the eleventh chapter he makes the following request:

> From Thee, Krishna of the lotus eyes, I have heard at length of the origin and dissolution of beings, as also of Thy inexhaustible greatness.
>
> So it is, O Krishna, as Thou hast declared Thyself, still I desire to see Thy Ishvara-Form.

Ishvara-Form means Krishna's Divine form. Arjuna is by this time convinced of his teacher's wisdom but still displays a very human curiosity to see everything for himself. Krishna thereupon replies:

> But thou canst not see Me with these mortal eyes of thine, Arjuna. Therefore I give thee supersensuous sight. Now behold my Yoga Power Supreme.

It would not be possible to understand the full meaning of the Gita, or indeed any other great poem, by a cold, analytical approach. To do full justice to a work of Art one must *experience* it, and to experience the Gita is to share the vision of Arjuna at this shattering moment.

> If the light of a thousand suns were to rise up at once in the sky, that splendour might be compared with the radiance of Thy Mighty Being.

Trembling, and with his palms joined together, he prostrates himself before Krishna and speaks in a choked voice, hardly able to express what he feels at that moment. He tells his Lord in the follow-

56

ing passage that he is appalled by his former treatment of Krishna as a friend and equal:

> Whatever I have presumptuously said from carelessness or love, addressing Thee as 'Krishna, Yadava, and friend', regarding Thee merely as a friend, unconscious of this Thy Greatness—in whatever way I may have been disrespectful to Thee; often I would jest as we walked, ate, rested together, alone or in company. Have I offended Thee? If this is so, then I ask your forgiveness.

Krishna replies in words to be found in the Bible of Judaism and Christianity: 'Be not afraid'.

Henceforth, of course, there is no longer any duality in Arjuna's attitude towards Krishna. He becomes, at last, One with his Lord. Having examined this relationship at some length, we can now return to the beginning of the Gita in which we find Arjuna in a dilemma which is at once human and universal. We follow his progress through the Gita as with the aid of Krishna, and making many mistakes on the way, he evolves from the darkness of ignorance into a region,

> Made radiant by the luminous lamp of Knowledge,

and Knowledge is the theme of the second chapter, in which Krishna explains to Arjuna the basic principles of Karma Yoga. All action, all work, if performed in the spirit of joy and selflessness, can lead to harmony in a man's mind, and harmony between his lower and his Higher Self. Karma Yoga is wisdom in work but I would point out here that the sages of ancient India were by no means alone in this viewpoint.

Homer, the great poet of ancient Greece writes of work as being both inherently beautiful and therapeutic and we can find this very same concept of the value of work in many of the great literary masterpieces of the world. In the Apocryphal New Testament—to quote but one example—are the words:

> Let the wise man show forth his wisdom, not in words but in good works.

Indeed doctors in modern hospitals, particularly in mental hospitals, now understand well the therapeutic value of work, and countless patients have accordingly benefited from occupational therapy. Karma Yoga is nothing if not sound common sense!

The subject of Karma Yoga recurs throughout the Gita after this second chapter, and in the third to the sixth chapters it is discussed in ever greater detail together with Jnana Yoga, the great Yoga of Knowledge, and reference is made also to Bhakti, the Yoga of the meditative. There is an interesting verse in Chapter Four in which Sri Krishna answers a question which Man has been asking since time immemorial. The verse reads:

> In whatever way men worship Me, in the same way do I fulfil their desires; it is My path, Arjuna, that men tread in all their ways.

The interpretation of this verse is as follows. Some people object that God appears to favour some men more than others, and some not at all. Some men are blessed with wisdom and Self-Knowledge, while the minds of others, clouded with the darkness of delusion, are never at peace. Krishna makes it clear that this apparent discrepancy is in no way due to any partiality in God's attitude towards men; that on the contrary, the difference is due to the differing attitudes of men towards Him; and that the *choice* is entirely up to them. Krishna makes it clear in the following verse that because worldly success is far easier to attain than Self-Knowledge, most men try for the former, and he declares that in so doing they are acting from ignorance. He tells Arjuna further on that even wise men are sometimes bewildered as to the meaning of inaction, and action in inaction, and clarifies these cryptic phrases in unequivocal terms.

In the fifth chapter, in verses 14 and 15, the Gita elucidates the relationship of God to the Universe:

> 14. No action does the Lord create for the Universe, nor does He bring about the result of action. Universal ignorance is alone the cause.
> 15. The All-Knowing recognizes neither the merit nor the demerit of any man. Knowledge is enveloped in ignorance, hence do men become deluded.

The entire teaching of the Bhagavad Gita, indeed of the whole Hindu scriptures, is condensed into these two verses which can be summed up as follows. That the Lord is perfect and without motive because such would be contrary to His nature. But His proximity to Nature invests the latter with the power of cause and effect. The individual being, which in the Gita is called Jiva, is in bondage so long as he identifies himself with Nature (cause and effect) instead of the God-head behind it.

In Chapter Six Arjuna protests that he does not see the possibility of lasting peace because of the restless nature of the mind.

'Verily the mind, O Krishna,' he says, 'is restless, turbulent, strong and unyielding, as hard to control as the wind.'

Krishna quite understands Arjuna's objection and answers him with the following words:

Without doubt, Arjuna, the mind is restless and difficult to bring under control. This can only be done by constant practice.

But Arjuna is still doubtful.

If a man strives and fails, Krishna, and his mind wanders away from Yoga, what is his end? Does he not, fallen from both the paths of knowledge and action, far from earth and far from heaven, tossed by the pathless winds, without support, Krishna, does he not perish?

To help my readers to understand Krishna's reply to this, I must point out that the Vedic ideal is to be freed from the cycle of birth and death, that the man who is able to achieve union (Yoga) with Brahman, the Absolute, is not born again, for to be born is to be fettered by the bodily self, and the upward struggle has to begin all over again. Krishna's reply is as follows:

Having attained to the worlds of the righteous, one fallen from Yoga does not perish. He dwells for many years among the right-eous, and then is born again into a family of wise Yogis, into a house where the wisdom of Yoga shines. Such a birth is rare in this world, Arjuna, because this man begins his new life armed with the wisdom of his former life. But still he must strive, and perchance through many lives to come, but in the end he will attain perfection.

In the seventh chapter Krishna describes His own nature and in so doing reveals the pantheistic doctrine of the Vedanta. Philosophy and poetry are welded together here and the result is profound and awesome:

> I am the sapidity in water, O Arjuna,
> I the radiance in the moon and sun,
> I am the OM in all the Vedas
> and the manhood in men.
>
> I am the sweet fragrance in earth
> and the brilliance in fire am I,
> the Life in all beings
> and the austerity am I in ascetics.

The poetry of this seventh chapter is so ravishing that it has clearly transcended all barriers of language.

> Know me, O son of Pritha
> as the eternal seed of all life,
> I am the intellect of the intelligent
> the heroism of the heroic.
> Of the strong I am the strength . . .

Krishna goes on to explain to Arjuna that most people in the world are unable to grasp this concept of the divine in all things, that the quintessence of all things is that which is called God. Men are deluded by their emotions (as Arjuna himself was at the beginning of the dialogue), and only the man with clarity of vision, a rare being, is able to understand. Krishna is well aware of how difficult this can be.

He then tells Arjuna of the four kinds of men who, purified by their good deeds, worship Him: the man who is weary of the world, the man who seeks knowledge, he who looks for real peace of mind, and the man who is blessed with spiritual discrimination. Of these four types, the last is the highest and therefore nearest to Brahman. Krishna continues:

> I am not manifest to all,
> being veiled by My mysterious power,
> This ignorant world knows Me not.

The great Yoga teacher, Swami Vivekananda, regarded ignorance as the cause of all the distress and evil in the world, and although many thinking people have closely examined his argument, none has ever succeeded in refuting it. In the Gita it is repeatedly shown that the state of ignorance is the enemy of Yoga, but that *awareness* of ignorance is the beginning of knowledge.

No knowledge of the Self has the man of ignorance, nor has he meditation. To the one who has not meditation there is no peace. And how can one without peace attain happiness, Arjuna? . . .

For the mind, which follows in the wake of the wandering senses, carries away his discrimination, as a wind carries away from its course a ship on the ocean . . .

The illumined soul must not create confusion in the minds of ignorant men by refraining from action. The wise man, himself steadily acting, should engage the ignorant in all works . . .

Without Brahman a man is in bondage,
enslaved by action and the desire for its fruits,
he dreams he is the doer, entitled to the fruits of his deeds.
God gives not this delusion, it is universal ignorance . . .

The evil-doers and the deluded are the lowest of men,
Deprived of discrimination by Maya [delusion]
They devote not themselves to Me, but follow the way of
    ignorance . . .

The ignorant regard me, Arjuna, as come into manifestation,
not knowing My supreme state, immutable and transcendental . . .

Unaware of My higher state, as the great Lord of beings, fools disregard Me, dwelling in the human form . . .

Even those who worship other deities with true faith
Worship Me alone, O Arjuna, but mistakenly, and not in the way they can find Moksha [Liberation] . . .

Krishna tells Arjuna that He is like fire which gives heat to all who draw near to it, but not to those who move away from it. And like sunlight, which is reflected in a clean mirror, He can be seen only by the wise, in other words by those from whose minds all the grime of ignorance has been cleared away.

The music of the Gita continues, and new themes are interwoven with those already introduced—that of unchanging love, and the concept of the mind being above the senses, the latter being introduced as early as the third chapter in which Krishna says:

> The senses are said to be superior to the body; the mind is superior to the senses; the intellect is superior to the mind; and that which is superior to the intellect is Brahman (The Self).

Having heard something of Krishna's nature (Chapter Seven) we find Arjuna insatiable, eager to hear more. In the tenth chapter he says to Krishna,

> Speak to me again in detail, O Krishna, of Thy Yoga Powers and attributes, for I am never satisfied in hearing of them, and of Thy speech.

So Krishna goes on to tell Arjuna of His divine attributes in the following words:

> I am the Self in the heart of all things, I am the beginning, the middle, and also the end of all beings.
> I am the radiant sun and the winds and the light of the moon . . .
> Of waters I am the oceans, of immovable things I am the Himalayas.
> I am trees and animals, and of men the king.

He then goes on to describe his terrible aspect with the same poetic force as his benevolence and his divinity.

> Of weapons I am the thunderbolt, I am serpents and water-beings,
> Of measures I am Time, and of fishes the shark . . .
> I am the all-destroying death.
> Of punishers I am the sceptre.
> There is no end of my divine attributes, Arjuna, and this is but a brief statement to thee.

Krishna has yet another aspect which he describes in the tenth chapter.

Of feminine nouns I am fame, beauty, prosperity,
Inspiration, memory, intelligence,
constancy and patient forgiveness.
Of the seasons, I am the season of flowers . . .

This chapter ends with Krishna asking Arjuna,

But why need you, Arjuna, to know all this diversity?
Know thou this only, that I exist, supporting this whole universe
by a single atom of Myself.

At the beginning of the eleventh chapter we find Arjuna, though no longer doubting Krishna's words, yet still displaying a very human curiosity to see all this splendour for himself. Krishna complies.

Arjuna is dazzled and terrified, as any mortal would be in such a situation. He bows low, and speaks to Krishna in a voice choking with fear and wonder,

O Krishna, if a thousand suns were to rise up at once into the sky,
that would be like the splendour of Thy mighty Form.
I see Thee with diadem, club and discus,
A mass of radiance shining everywhere, dazzling my eyes, striking fear into all worlds,
And I also, I also am afraid.

And because no mortal could endure such a sight for any length of time, Arjuna begs Krishna to assume, once more, his human form with which he (Arjuna) is so familiar. So Krishna appears in his former shape and,

Assuming once more his mild and pleasing form, calmed the fears and brought peace to him who was terrified.

Arjuna is vastly relieved.

O Krishna, now I see Thy gentle human form, my thoughts are now composed, I am myself once more.

The twelfth chapter is a treatise on Bhakti Yoga and in most translations is entitled, 'The Yoga of Devotion' or 'The Way of Devotion'. Krishna explains that there are two ways of practising this Yoga, one less difficult than the other as a concession to human fallibility. But above all, Krishna says, a man should not hate any living creature and must, at all times, be both friendly and compassionate. He must be dependent on no person and must treat friends and foes equally. He must be content with anything, even if he has no home.

Obviously this is a way of life which would be impossible to follow in our Western society but we must remember that the disciplines documented in the Gita are an *ideal* by which we may all aim our endeavours. Krishna is aware that most ordinary mortals do not, indeed cannot reach this high standard, and he says so in the seventh chapter:

> One, perchance, among thousands of men, strives for perfection;
> And one, perchance among these attains it.
> Such a one is the rarest of men.

The thirteenth to the eighteenth chapters of the Gita form the third and final section of the book. The thirteenth is a discussion of the human body and its relationship to its higher Self. The main theme of this chapter is that Yoga or union with the higher Self is the only way to attain everlasting Peace and it is separation of the lower and higher selves, or in other words, the sense of individuality, which is the cause of all our experiences of pleasure and pain. Krishna points out that:

> This Truth has been sung by Rishis [Seers of Truth] in many ways,
> In various distinctive chants, in aphorisms on the nature of Brahman,
> Subtly reasoned, wholly convincing.

To give but one or two examples of this subtle and convincing reasoning I will quote the following:

> Whenever a man coveteth anything inordinately, he is presently disquieted in himself. The proud and covetous are never at rest; the poor and humble in spirit dwell in abundance of peace. The

man that is not yet perfectly dead to himself is soon tempted and overcome in small and mean things. He that is weak in spirit and still in a measure prone to things of sense, can hardly withdraw himself altogether from earthly desires. And therefore oftentimes when he withdraweth from them he is sad, and he is readily moved to anger if any man withstandeth him. And if he obtain that which he desires he is presently stricken with remorse of conscience, for that he hath followed his own passion, which helpeth nothing to the peace that he sought. In withstanding the wishes of the senses, therefore, and not in obeying them, is found true peace of heart.

Thomas À Kempis

In this present life, I reckon that we make the nearest approach to knowledge when we have the least possible communion with the body, and are not contaminated with the bodily nature, but keep ourselves pure until the hour when God himself is pleased to release us.

When the soul uses the body as an instrument of perception, that is to say, when it uses the sense of sight or hearing or some other sense, she is dragged by the body into the region of the changeable, and wanders and is confused; the world spins round her, and she is like a drunkard, when she touches change. But when she contemplates in herself and by herself, then she passes into the other world, the region of purity, and eternity, and immortality, and unchangeableness, which are her kindred, and with them she ever lives, when she is by herself . . . then she ceases from her erring ways and being in communion with the unchanging is herself unchanging. And this state of soul is called wisdom.

Plato Phaedo

Since my dear soul was mistress of her choice,
And could of men distinguish, her election
Hath seal'd thee for herself: for thou hast been
As one, in suffering all, that suffers nothing;
A man that fortune's buffets and rewards
Hast ta'en with equal thanks: and blest are those
Whose blood and judgement are so well commingled,
That they are not a pipe for fortune's finger
To sound what stop she please. Give me that man

65

That is not passion's slave, and I will wear him
In my heart's core, ay, in my heart of heart,
As I do thee.

SHAKESPEARE Hamlet

The fourteenth chapter of the Gita explains the three Gunas which I have already discussed in Question 9 of the first chapter of this book. Krishna tells Arjuna that on the way to Brahman a man must be aware of the three Gunas, learn not to hate them, and thus go beyond them.

> The same in honour and dishonour, the same to friend and foe, relinquishing all undertakings—he, Arjuna, is said to have gone beyond the Gunas.
> And he who serves Me with unswerving devotion, he, going beyond the Gunas, is fitted to be One with Brahman.

In Chapter Fifteen Krishna tells Arjuna of the ancient story of a fig tree, a giant tree called Ashvattha, whose roots are in Heaven and its branches towards the earth. Each of its leaves is one of the songs of the Vedas.

> Below and above spread its branches, nourished by the Gunas; Sense-objects are its buds; and below in the world of man also stretch forth its roots, originating action.
> Its form is not here perceived as such, neither its end, nor its origin, nor its existence . . .

Man must, with the sharp axe of non-attachment, says Krishna, cut through this firm-rooted tree before he can go beyond Samsara (the world of change or the relative world). He must try then to return to that Primal State from which there is no return to future births.

This rather obscure passage in the Gita may be more easily understood if one reads the following extract from Wordsworth's Ode, *Intimations of Immortality*:

> Our birth is but a sleep and a forgetting:
> The Soul that rises with us, our life's Star,
> Hath had elsewhere its setting,
> And cometh from afar:

And not in utter nakedness,
Not in entire forgetfulness,
But trailing clouds of glory do we come
From God, who is our home:
Heaven lies about us in our infancy!

Shades of the prison-house begin to close
Upon the growing Boy,
But He beholds the light, and whence it flows,
He sees it in his joy;
The Youth, who daily farther from the east
Must travel, still in Nature's Priest,
And by the vision splendid
Is on his way attended;
At length the Man perceives it die away,
And fade into the light of common day.

This, of course, is a statement of the human predicament, the remedy for which is suggested in the Gita. Krishna tells Arjuna:

I am centred in the hearts of all; memory and perception as well as their loss come from Me.

Krishna continues further on thus:

As I transcend the Perishable [that is the giant fig tree called Ashvattha] and am above even the Imperishable, therefore am I in the world and also in the Vedas celebrated as the Highest Self . . . Knowing this one attains the highest intelligence and will have accomplished all one's duties, O Arjuna.

With these words the fifteenth chapter ends.

The sixteenth examines the two types of men to be found in the world: those whose nature tends towards the upward way, and those who have demonic tendencies. Having told Arjuna at length about the former, Krishna now turns his attention to those whom he calls 'persons of the Asurika nature'.

These persons know not what to do and from what to refrain; neither is purity found in them nor good conduct, nor truth. They say that the universe is without truth, without moral law, without a God.

Holding this view, these ruined souls of small intellect and fierce deeds, rise as the enemies of the world for its destruction. Filled with insatiable desires, full of hypocrisy, pride and arrogance, holding evil ideas through delusion, they work with impure resolve.

Beset with immense cares ending only with death, regarding gratification of the senses as the highest, they feel sure that this is all.

These malicious and cruel evil-doers, Krishna says, are perpetually reborn as evil beings such as tigers and snakes, not even men at all. To avoid such a hell as this, the ruin of the Self, Man must avoid three dark doors—lust, anger and greed. Let him beware, then, of flouting the scriptures.

The seventeenth chapter finds Arjuna telling Krishna that many men do not follow the teaching of the scriptures but are nevertheless men of faith. What then, he asks, is the nature of that faith? Krishna replies that the faith of each individual corresponds to his particular temperament, and whatsoever his temperament may be, so is his faith. These men fall into three types, and Krishna goes on to describe each in turn. This chapter explodes many of the senseless myths that have grown up around Yoga.

The eighteenth and last chapter of the Gita answers a question that has puzzled many of my own pupils, namely, what is the real meaning of renunciation and non-attachment and is there any difference between these two principles and if so, what are they? Krishna replies at length but a summing-up of his words is that it is the *ego* which has to be renounced.

He who is free from the notion of egoism, whose intelligence is not affected by good or evil. . . .

He whose consciousness of self is not confused or identified with the body or the mind, even when performing physical actions, he is forever free from the taint of delusion.

Of non-attachment he says:

The well-poised, forsaking the fruit of action, attains peace. The unbalanced one, led by the desire for the fruits of his actions,

68

is in bondage.

My own Guru used to tell me that the way to *live* Yoga is to do things for no other reason than that they need to be done. In other words to perform actions when they seem right and necessary but without any thought of oneself. If one performs actions in this way for long enough, thanks become a positive embarrassment. I have found this to be so.

The final part of the Gita sums up the whole work. Krishna tells Arjuna about the three kinds of happiness available to mankind. These arise from the three Gunas from whom no mortal is free because the Gunas come forth from Prakriti (Primordial Nature). So each individual may become perfect if he performs the work natural to his particular nature, and even if this work is done imperfectly, it is far better than any attempt to do work which is not natural to him. In any case, Krishna points out, it is as impossible to separate action from imperfection as to separate smoke from fire. This is put very succinctly in the following two verses:

Better is one's own duty, though imperfect, than the duty of another well performed. He who does the duty ordained by his own nature incurs no evil.

One should not relinquish, O Arjuna, the duty to which one is born, though it is attended with evil; for all undertakings are enveloped by evil, as fire by smoke.

Krishna reiterates his warning to Arjuna about egoism, power, pride, lust, wrath and property:

Freed from the notion of 'mine', and tranquil;—he alone is fit to be One with Brahman ...

Thus has wisdom, more profound than all profundities, been declared to thee, Arjuna, by Me; reflecting over it fully, act as thou thinkest best ...

But beware, Arjuna, you must never tell My words to anyone who lacks faith, devotion and self-control, or to one who disobeys his teacher, or who mocks at God. Tell it to no man who does not wish to hear it.

Krishna goes on further to ask Arjuna:

> Hast this been heard by thee with an attentive mind? Has the delusion of thy ignorance been destroyed?

Arjuna replies that indeed it has and that all his doubts have been dispelled. In other words, he has discovered that the true purpose of his life has been fulfilled and he has recognized his real Self.

The teaching of the Gita virtually ends here. The rest of the book serves to re-connect it with the main narrative, that is with the Mahabharata.

Sanjaya, upon whom the sage Vyasa (traditionally supposed to be the author of the Gita) has bestowed special powers of clairvoyance and clairaudience in order that he may witness the dialogue between Krishna and Arjuna and thereby report it to the blind King Dhritarashtra, then says:

> Thus have I heard this dialogue between Lord Krishna and the high-souled Arjuna, causing my hair to stand on end. Through the grace of Vyasa have I heard this supreme and profound Yoga, direct from Lord Krishna, Lord of Yoga, Himself declaring it.
>
> Wherever is Krishna, the Lord of Yoga, and wherever is Arjuna, the warrior Prince, wielder of the bow, there are prosperity, victory, triumph and glory; such is my conviction.

Thus ends the Shrimad-Bhagavad-Gita, which incorporates the Essence of the Upanishads, the Knowledge of Brahman, and the philosophy of Yoga.

OM! Peace! Peace! Peace!

Chapter 3

YOGA IN EVERYDAY LIFE

Quocirca vivite fortes,
Fortiaque adversis opponite pectora rebus
—On that account live as brave men, and
oppose brave hearts to adverse fate.

HORACE

THERE is a story about the two seas of Israel. One sea is filled with
fresh and sparkling water; it teems with fish and its banks are lush
with fruitful life. Jesus, it is said, loved this sea whose waters are
carried down by the River Jordan, and some of His happiest hours
were spent upon its shores.

But the Jordan also flows into another sea where there is no life
and whose banks are desert. The air above it is heavy and menacing;
fish do not live in it and neither man nor beast will drink its waters.
Why are these two seas of Israel so different? Because the beautiful
Sea of Galilee receives, but does not keep, the waters of the Jordan,
and the more it gives to the sea the more it receives from the river.
The Sea of Galilee is the Sea of Life. But the other, aptly named the
Dead Sea, hoards every drop of water which flows into it and gives
none away. It gives nothing and does not live.

Life works this way with people. The happiest ones are the givers,
those who are not afraid to give their concern for their fellow men,
their love, their compassion, their time, their energy towards making
the lives of others easier. The miserable ones are the selfish ones,
the misers, the misanthropes. Money need not come into it. You can
be a miser with your feelings, your time, your hospitality, your willingness to do someone a good turn.

What might be termed a normal happy life is neither more nor
less than a courageous approach to life and its day-to-day problems,
and a wisely objective solution to these problems as and when they
arise.

The person who wishes to incorporate Yoga into his everyday life, and thereby find a greater sense of peace and fulfilment, will find it necessary to cultivate four quintessential elements.

Firstly an awareness of other people and their needs. Secondly compassion, hospitality and generosity towards his fellow men and a willingness to contribute to the common weal in terms of useful work. Thirdly a sense of humour and fourthly the application of the other three to his everyday life, in other words maintaining a zest for life in spite of all its vicissitudes. This requires a high degree of courage but the results to be gained correlate to that courage in exact proportion.

Every living organism makes its own characteristic response to the challenge of existence to secure the maintenance of life, and Man is no exception. His characteristic solution is the formation of social groups and communities. Society is his line of defence against the forces of nature. It therefore follows logically that a fulfilled human being must be a member of a group. The converse is also true; a human being who is physically, mentally and emotionally isolated is lonely and miserable.

This brings me to another truth of paramount importance in human existence and that is the value of work. Society exists for the protection of the individual but requires of every individual a contribution towards the maintenance of the group. Work is one of the primary sources of personal salvation (I refer my readers to the chapter on Karma Yoga in this book), work being as vitally important as social adjustment.

It therefore follows that any individual who does not solve the problems of existence in a socially acceptable manner is liable to feel exposed to the dangers of an unfriendly world. This in turn gives rise to anxiety, fear, and a sense of personal inadequacy. In Yoga this approach to life would be considered a 'bad life technique'. Think of it this way. If you suffer from a sense of personal inadequacy it indicates that you are basing your life on a fallacy. A simple analogy will clarify this. You believe you can win security and happiness by building walls round yourself rather than by building bridges to your fellow men.

Which brings me to another important point in this discussion of Yoga in everyday life and that is inter-personal relationships. Some people, when they are alone, feel strong and whole, completely in charge of themselves. At such times they are at peace, but as soon as they come into contact with other people they find themselves diminished as individuals. Suddenly they become confused and lose self-confidence. These people are often students of Yoga who, having attained some measure of peace of mind, suddenly find themselves in the company of people who are not, as I call it, 'Yoga minded'. The problem is how does the sensitive, thinking person, often a student of Yoga, cope with those who are out of sympathy with his convictions, and way of life?

One of the aims of Yoga is to develop the personality, the uniqueness of the individual, to its highest potential. The student of Yoga must therefore strive to overcome the negative pull-back caused by other people, and learn to protect himself from alien influences. Left to ourselves we would all make unhampered progress towards perfect harmony of mind and body, and achieve that calmness and balance that is the hall-mark of every enlightened person. But in the 1970s we are surrounded by more and more people and the challenge becomes more formidable every day.

The way of Yoga is always strewn with rocks that impede progress, yet to the determined person no obstacle is insurmountable. This is a truth that can be applied to everyone striving to achieve something, whether it be mastery of Yoga or anything else.

Having then taken up the challenge of these other people who seem to sap our inner strength, and recognizing them as an obstacle to be surmounted—and nothing more than that—we have already reduced them in size. If we allow them to grow large in our minds they will loom and dominate. So I want to approach this obstacle in two ways, the negative and then the positive. By negative I mean that if other people are your problem then you must learn how to *protect* yourself against them. Having learned to do this you are then ready to take a more positive attitude towards the relationships between yourself and other people; in other words you will then be able to communicate with your fellow beings on your own terms and not as a diminished personality.

There is an exercise for protecting yourself which you can practise any time you feel another person's alien vibrations hit you. Sit or stand still and join your first finger and thumb to 'seal in' your prana or inner power. Do this with both hands. It can be done quite unobtrusively wherever you may be. Having done this imagine you are sitting (or standing) inside a large and transparent egg. You are able to see and hear everything around you, but inside your 'egg' you are safe from negative or alien vibrations. This is a good exercise to practise every day because when it becomes second nature your egg will be there automatically protecting you whenever you feel you need it.

Having mastered this exercise you can take it a step further. From inside your protective shell take a long hard look at the person who distresses you or tries to diminish you. From where you are you will be able to see this person objectively, as an ordinary human being instead of a kind of monster.

It is very easy, when we dislike or are afraid of someone, or feel uneasy in their company, to regard them as larger than life, so it is important to be able to bring them down to our own size. They are much more manageable that way.

This mental exercise becomes easier the more you practise it but it will help you to be objective about people and once you can be so with regard to those who distress you, you will never be diminished or inhibited about them again. Or to put it another way, if you are diminished by another person it is because you are emotionally involved, you are afraid of what they will think. If this is the basis of the relationship between you, then the personality of the other person will naturally dominate yours.

So free yourself from this involvement by practising objectivity and in time your own personality will expand and assert itself and you will no longer feel shy or afraid or inhibited with others. This in turn will have its effect on others because if your own nature expands and asserts itself freely when in the company of others, they will no longer regard you, and therefore treat you, in such a way as to make you feel at a disadvantage.

Having liberated your own personality, there remains the positive approach to other people. This involves another mental exercise. First you need a 'peace symbol'—I always use a white rose but anything which is essentially beautiful and still would be appropriate. Sit quietly and close your eyes, training your mind on whatever you are using as a peace symbol. Try to still all circling thoughts or if you cannot do this, keep leading your mind deliberately back to your symbol until your thoughts begin to slow down. Open your eyes at this point, *without moving your head*, and look about you as far as you can.

When you have explored everything within this narrow field of vision you can then turn your head and look at everything around you. You will, for a few seconds, experience a sense of heightened awareness, colours will be brighter and have more depth, textures will be richer, you will hear sounds more acutely, your senses will literally be more acute.

The idea behind this exercise is as follows: Once the mind is as still as possible and uncluttered by negative emotion, pre-conceived ideas or prejudice and so on, it can function as a more efficient instrument on a level which will enable you to be aware of things as they are and not as you *think* they are.

This also applies to people, which is even more important to you in your everyday life. Practise the exercise when in the company of other people and you will soon be able to see further than their persona, which is the image they project, their worldly face if you like. You will be able to see 'into' people if you train your mind to a state of heightened awareness by means of this exercise.

It is always of vital importance to know the sort of person you are dealing with. It is useful to know whom you can trust and whom you cannot. It is useful to know if this man or woman is going to be reasonable or otherwise as a boss, a landlord, an M.P., a teacher or any other kind of person whom you may need. It makes life easier if you know, instead of just guessing, what another person is like. And it is useful to find out (and not the hard way!) who your real friends are.

The above is the common sense way of discussing what in the Bhagavad Gita is called Maya or illusion. One reads of 'the darkness of Maya'.

Lord Krishna says to Arjuna,

Thinking of objects, attachment to them is formed in a man. From attachment there comes longing, and from longing anger grows. From anger comes Maya [illusion or delusion], and from Maya there comes loss of memory. From loss of memory there comes the ruin of discrimination.

Many of my pupils have questioned the logic of the words—'from longing anger grows' so I will clarify this. Let us imagine a man sitting down to clear his mind of circling thoughts in order to achieve the state of heightened awareness. An image comes to his mind, and if this image is something beautiful the tendency of his mind will be to dwell on it. With this recurring image there gradually comes a wish to possess. If it is something which he knows he can never possess, then resentment will enter his mind and grow there. This in its turn will produce anger which throws the mind into confusion, and this will be a bar to his achievement of a heightened sense of awareness. So he will have to begin the mental exercise all over again. So Krishna warns Arjuna not to let any insidious thoughts enter his mind lest they cause him to think, and subsequently act, irrationally.

But with constant practice you can perfect these two mental disciplines and life will consequently present fewer problems in respect of inter-personal relationships, whether casual or of a closer nature. But there is another problem with which Man is faced in the 1970s. Technology has placed in the hands of Man a vast amount of power which has been derived from the control of the forces of nature. While the control of this power has greatly increased the material well-being of man, it has disturbed the comparatively static human situation of centuries. And out of what has become an intensified social mobility has come a situation in which instability and insecurity are prevalent.

If you are one of those people who suffer from this particular human predicament and feel that Yoga is an effective antidote, then there are four stages by means of which you can live in the world and yet feel whole and at peace with yourself. The four stages are as follows:

1. *Learn to know yourself*. You can do this by being absolutely honest with yourself about your feelings, motivations, intentions, and so on. You need not share this painful process with anyone else. Ruthless honesty with oneself is a prerequisite of Yoga and is seldom a pleasant phase to go through. You will find at first that you are not quite the person you thought you were. You might even be shocked at your discoveries about yourself, but this is part of the discipline and no one who wants to study Yoga should shirk this stage of the proceedings.

2. Having learned about yourself the idea is to *modify your character into something meaningful*, something that you yourself would respect and admire. Read the Bhagavad Gita and in its pages you will learn the means by which you can become whatever sort of person you wish to be.

3. Having learned to know yourself and having made your character more positive, you will have to plan your time carefully so that you *live your life to its fullest extent*. Do something you have

76

always wanted to do. Do not just talk about it, that wastes time. Plan your campaign and then act on it. You will find you are really living instead of just existing.

4. *Learn not to be daunted by obstacles.* If you think of Yoga as four paths, then I can tell you they are all strewn with boulders. Every discipline interposes obstacles in the way of the aspirant. Learn to take these as they come. Do not anticipate them but work quietly until you come up against a problem. Then use your sense of logic to work out the best solution. This is a fine discipline for the mind, and you will find that by performing the above four disciplines you will find everyday life not a burden, but an adventure.

Chapter 4

INTER-PERSONAL RELATIONSHIPS

The man who can do without his fellows is either a beast or a god.
ARISTOTLE

HUMAN relationships were once described by Professor John Mac-murray as being of three kinds: instrumental, organic and personal.

1. An instrumental relationship is one in which one person regards and uses another as a means to an end or as an instrument by means of which he may achieve some desired end.

2. An organic relationship occurs when both members belong to a group. The purpose of this type of relationship is the promotion of some common interest.

3. A personal relationship exists for its own sake though both parties need a common interest or purpose through which to express the relationship which otherwise would come to an inevitable end.

It may surprise many people who are reading about inter-personal relationships for the first time that any one of the above three kinds may lie at the heart of the most important relationship of our adult years, namely marriage.

Four distinct but common types of disruptive conflict occur in relationships: dependency, domination, hostility and indifference. *Dependency* is found in practically every marriage. We are, as a species, interdependent and what is important is the degree of dependency and its effects on inter-personal relationships. This dependency manifests itself in different ways. Some people have little capacity to stand on their own feet, and this may manifest itself in the form of jealousy or possessiveness, or in excessive demands on the partner. On the other hand the person who is so heavily leaned on usually needs a period of adjustment at the outset of the relationship to learn the acceptance of being a prop. To show impatience or open hostility may reduce the dependent person to despair which will put a great degree of strain on the relationship.

Domination is one of the primary causes of conflict in relationships.

Though the dominating partner may rationalize his or her behaviour in some way, it does have the inevitable tendency to arouse hostile reactions in the dominated person. It is therefore of vital importance to understand that behind any attitudes of domination lie feelings of personal inadequacy or inferiority, and other neurotic convictions. In some cases both parties in a relationship may be guilty of domination, the initially dominated person guarding his own personality from being overwhelmed by reacting in a like manner to dictatorial behaviour.

Some manifestations of this type of behaviour are obvious: aggression in the form of shouting, tyranny, violence, physical and mental cruelty. Others are less obvious: nagging, sulking, touchiness, or even physical or emotional disorders.

Hostility is a universal human emotion and there is some element of it in every relationship. Some people who enter into a relationship with fairy-tale expectations of living 'happily ever after' may be frightened of, or disillusioned by, the first manifestations of hostility. It is therefore of great importance to remind oneself from time to time of the universality of hostility and to accept it for what it is, attaching no great significance to it except in so far as it may threaten the stability of the relationship.

Some of the manifestations of hostility are constant and unnecessary criticism, sarcasm, slander, disloyalty, sulking, constantly putting blame on the other party, belittling, sneering, malicious behaviour, physical and mental violence and cruelty. Often conflicts in relationships arise because of personal differences which neither party can understand, accept or tolerate, due to a lack of maturity. If possible the presence of conflict should be faced and the causes examined by both parties before the relationship becomes seriously undermined and eventually breaks down.

The fourth type of disruptive conflict which can occur in relationships is indifference. This is like a slow disease which manifests itself in different ways: a lack of interest in or awareness of the needs of the other person; neglect of the essential co-operation required to keep the relationship alive; lack of any real communication between the parties. Indifference is a more serious disorder of relationships than hostility, being less overt, more insidious and therefore that much more difficult to diagnose. The opposite of indifference is an enthusiasm for the relationship which provides the necessary motivation and the sustaining bond.

When indifference invades a relationship the deep-rooted needs of the parties for affection, companionship and acceptance are frustrated, and this creates the kind of atmosphere in which the relationship is likely to disintegrate. Indifference occurs for a variety of reasons: the fact of the relationships being based on inadequate foundations, both parties having personal inadequacies, a lack of understanding, or overwhelming pressures of environment. If both sides wish to save a relationship which has been affected by indifference it is necessary for all possible factors to be faced, examined and accepted so that they may be tackled as problems. It is then necessary for both parties to try to discover as many of the background reasons as possible, because only when the causative factors can be discovered and understood can a damaged relationship be saved.

Yoga's common sense method of dealing with difficulties in relationships is the dispelling of ignorance through the study and practice of Karma Yoga, the Yoga of cause and effect, the essentially *practical* Yoga which I discuss in Chapter Six of the present volume. This, together with careful reading of books and articles on the subject plus the guidance of an expert Yoga teacher, added to a great deal of patience and hard work can, in time, resolve difficulties. But the student of Yoga would do well to remember that no relationship can stand up to the strain of neglect. A relationship to be satisfactory to both parties has to be carefully tended just as anything which grows needs tending if it is to flourish. The main enemies of any relationship are intolerance, indifference, suspicion, lack of sensitivity and lack of maturity with which I will deal in some detail.

It must also be understood, though, that there are some environmental factors which can contribute to the breakdown of a relationship. These may be physical, personal, social, cultural or spiritual.

1. *Physical.* This encompasses housing and financial difficulties, personal possessions, lack of privacy, ill health etc.

2. *Personal.* Various interferences such as the disruptive influence of people outside the relationship, although in many cases of interference there is some underlying defect in the relationship which renders it vulnerable to outside pressures.

3. Under the heading of the *social and cultural* environment of relationships we can consider external environmental factors which can never be unrelated to social realities. These can be listed as follows: the emancipation of women, which has profoundly affected relationships; prevailing social ideas and practices in the community;

a lessening of emotional and intellectual communication due in part to the many complex technicalities of modern life.

It is often difficult for people conditioned to the highly competitive and aquisitive western world of the 1970s to re-orientate themselves to the mutual consideration and lack of selfishness which inter-personal relationships demand. This is why many people who are successful in the worldly sense are quite unable to maintain stable relationships.

The *spiritual* factor which I mentioned last has a strong influence on all kinds of relationships. This can be most easily explained by saying that the breakdown of many relationships is due to partners' having allowed selfish interests to take precedence over the mutual interests of the relationship. This can be due to no more no less than an absence of love or liking. These are most likely to be lacking when both partners in a relationship were brought up in an unstable back-ground—in particular an emotionally unstable background. I emphasize the word *likely* because by no means all, or even the majority of, people brought up in less than ideal conditions are unable to establish stable relationships later in life. Nevertheless the tendency remains for children with an unstable background to have some difficulty with inter-personal relationships later in life, in other words not to achieve mature relationships.

The ability to form satisfactory inter-personal relationships is one of the primary hall-marks of maturity. Others are the ability to live in harmony with society and the possession of a fully developed in-dividual character. The latter is necessary for the attainment of the first two, that is to say maturity represents in the first instance the fullest expression possible of the individual's innate potentialities. This can be achieved by means of Yoga or any other process which enables the individual to realize both his uniqueness as a person and his relationship to society.

Man is a gregarious animal and it is essential for each individual to realize and accept Man's need for other people. Few human beings are able to cope with themselves single-handed. It may, on the other hand, be argued that the uninterrupted development of the individual may conflict with the society in which he moves, and that a person can only be fully himself at the expense of other people. But it would seem that the basis of an adult's ability to establish satisfying and long-lasting relationships, and of adult self-confidence, is the sense of being *accepted* by other people without reservation. On the other

81

hand it is logical to deduce that the lack of balance in the personality which we call neurosis can be the result of lack of acceptance, either real or imaginary, in children so constituted as to have a predisposition towards neurosis.

Another aspect of maturity in inter-personal relationships is complete equality, that is to say the absence of domination on either side or any form of restriction which would provoke aggression, leading to fear and anxiety.

Individuals tend to identify with those people whom they like and who can be expected to evoke aspects of their personality which might otherwise remain dormant. This is the positive effect of identification. On the other hand, children tend to regard certain of their personality traits as undesirable and will try to suppress them. It is found, however, that in later life they will be disturbed by, and condemn, identical traits in other people, so long as they are unable to accept them in themselves.

The aspect of equality as a characteristic of truly mature inter-personal relationships is significant because in so many instances there is an element of passive receptivity on the one hand and dominance on the other. Many physically mature but emotionally immature people feel a sense of inferiority or inadequacy in relationships with other people and do not believe they have anything to contribute. These are the ones who regard others as being there to serve their needs, and consequently cannot establish any form of reciprocal relationship.

These unfortunate individuals live in a constant state of anxiety and dread—that is, dread of losing those upon whom they are dependent. Each person recognizes, subconsciously, his need of other people, and when the dread of losing love or friendship is present it is because the constantly developing personality structure is dependent upon sustained relationships with other individuals who not only accept one, 'warts and all', but by their continued presence give the reassurance one needs.

Those people who are in need of constant reassurance are not only emotionally immature but are actually incapable of sustaining balanced inter-personal relationships. This is because they are compelled to insist that their friends or loved ones conform, not to their own individual opinions, likes and dislikes, but to those of the immature individual. From this we can logically say that one of the most important signs of maturity is the ability to tolerate those different from oneself. A further sign is the individual's emotional establishment as a member of the sex to which he or she anatomically belongs, and more important still, the ability to *compete, on equal terms*, with others of the same sex.

A further important characteristic of mature relationships is the recognition that they are essentially progressive rather than static. Each party fulfils the other's needs but in addition each partner is regarded and treated by the other as a whole person. This is the state of equality to which I referred earlier, a state in which two people confront each other, each as an individual in his own right and without trying to alter the other.

One of the most important functions of Yoga is to help the individual towards maturity and all that it involves. This process is begun by establishing a dynamic and ever-changing relationship between the Yoga teacher and the student. At first the relationship can be tenuous when the teacher and student are, as it were, sizing each other up, the teacher because he or she is seeking to establish contact with the psychic life of the student, the latter because he or she is wondering what knowledge the teacher has to offer, whether that knowledge will enable the student to live a fuller, more varied, freer and more interesting life, and whether the study and practice of Yoga will offer a solution to his problems. At this stage the teacher stands in relation to the student as a parent figure, but after the initial stages when the student is, to a greater or lesser degree, dependent upon the teacher, the relationship becomes more evenly balanced. Finally the stage is reached when the relationship achieves solidarity, which can be said to exist when two individuals recognize each other on a basis of mutual understanding and respect.

The study of Yoga is of immense value in the process of maturing and the establishment of successful inter-personal relationships, because it is clear that the student's personality development and that of his relationships proceed side by side. In fact it is a psychological truth that the former cannot proceed without the latter. One might well argue, though, that Yoga does not offer anything which cannot be obtained through psycho-therapy. Up to a point this is true but after that I cannot agree. Many people who have problems of one sort or another feel at a disadvantage when seated facing a psychiatrist across a desk. Such a feeling can arouse fear and resentment because the therapeutic relationship is bound to be based to a greater or lesser degree on a situation of imbalance. The patient is seeking help and feels this keenly as he is confronted by the impassive face of the psychiatrist across the desk. Also (and this is not inconsiderable to a sensitive patient) there is the stigma attached to any form of emotional or mental disturbance, a stigma which persists in spite of the fact that this form of suffering is more prevalent in the West today than it has ever been. This social disadvantage could well be uppermost in the patient's mind when he first meets his psychiatrist and might give him a strong feeling of being at a disadvantage, no matter how well-trained and understanding the doctor might be.

On the other hand the Yoga teacher is much more acceptable to many over-sensitive people than the psychiatrist simply because the person seeking help knows he is not with a doctor. Lessons in Yoga are not, and should not, I think, be conducted in an atmosphere of formality as so many medical consultations are. The Yoga teacher sits near the pupil, usually on the floor, sometimes on a chair, and the pupil finds no difficulty in feeling at ease once the initial shyness has worn off. Yoga teachers have a reputation for being warmly human people and I have never yet met one who did not have a sense of humour. Indeed this humour can, and I believe should, be an important element in the relationship between teacher and student, not only because it promotes a feeling of informality but because the cultivation of a sense of humour is itself therapeutic. There is no easier way of establishing a bond between oneself and other individuals than to cultivate a genial personality. Also a sense of humour helps to lighten the burden of life by allowing the individual to see it as a kind of comic paradox.

I am reminded here of Oliver Goldsmith's work *Retaliation* (1774) in which he speaks of a man

who mixed reason with pleasure and wisdom with mirth;

and of Pope's *Essay on Criticism* (1711) in which he writes,

True wit is nature to advantage dressed,
What oft was thought, but ne'er so well expressed.

It is a well-known fact that humour is an attribute of those who feel reasonably at home in the world. To the person who is emotionally immature, sick, unhappy or afraid, laughter is a luxury he cannot afford. This is because no one can laugh when he is emotionally isolated from his fellows.

Humour plays an important part in inter-personal relationships;

84

in fact it is so successful a device for establishing greater solidarity between one human being and another that its importance can hardly be overestimated. And by humour I mean not only the ability to laugh at a good joke but the ability to laugh at ourselves so that we may go through life with courage and optimism, making the best of its harsh realities. Each one of us is infinitesimally small and frail and defenceless, in fact we are the weakest animals which inhabit the earth. At the same time we are the only living beings with the gift of humour, and this appreciation of the comical is a saving grace without which all thinking people would descend into depression and finally try to take their own lives.

It is therefore the duty of the Yoga teacher to help the student towards a healthier life, both physically and mentally. This implies the active use of innate human qualities such as the sense of humour, the sense of awareness, and a kindly and co-operative attitude towards others. It also implies complete utilization of all our senses, breadth of mind, and a healthy responsiveness to the most varied stimuli. These are the best insurance against the possibility of mental ill-health and that most paralysing of mind-states, a sense of futility.

The Yoga teacher has a further duty towards his student, namely he must help him to solve the not inconsiderable problem of utilizing his leisure. This was once a problem only to the wealthy. The machine age has made it the problem of the majority. The student of Yoga need not, and I believe should not, stop learning as long as he lives, not only about Yoga and philosophy in general but about anything and everything that captures his interest. To stop learning— and this means not only book learning—is to court mental atrophy. Not everyone has the desire for further education, but everyone has the need to utilize his mind. Mental energy can be directed towards a wide variety of different pursuits from social and welfare work to making model aeroplanes, gardening, or becoming expert at a game. It is up to the Yoga teacher to help the student to make the most useful, that is to say, health-promoting decisions in this matter. This is done by making the student aware of his own personality, his needs, wishes and capabilities (and equally important his limitations!) and then helping him towards the positive action to fulfil those needs etc. In all these and in other ways the teacher/student relationship is rewarding to both parties because it is ever evolving towards maturity. It is in fact a microcosm which reflects the macrocosm of their relationships outside the Yoga teacher's studio.

Chapter 5

SUFFERING

He's truly valiant, that can wisely suffer
The worst that man can breathe.
SHAKESPEARE *Timon of Athens*

ALL THINGS, animate and inanimate, are subject to the law of change. This of course includes the mind states. Happiness alternates with suffering, serenity with restlessness, exaltation with depression, anxiety and fear. And as change is a universal phenomenon, so too is suffering. Rich and poor alike, old and young, learned and illiterate, none can escape it.

The early philosophical writings of the Indo-Aryans refer to these two universal phenomena and throughout the centuries, until the present day, many philosophers have tended towards the belief that suffering is the price of being born.

Two thousand five hundred years ago the Buddha discovered four Truths which were to form the basis of his religion, and all four are related to suffering. They are as follows:

The elements which make up man produce a capacity for pain.
The cause of pain is the striving away from an embracing totality.
Deliverance from this striving causes pain to cease.
The way of deliverance is along the path of intuitive knowledge to the divine Source.

The Bhagavad Gita reiterates these four Truths in its own incomparable language:

The soul of man is his friend when by the Spirit he has conquered his soul, but when a man is not lord of his soul then this becomes his own enemy.

When the soul is at peace he is in peace, in cold and heat, pleasure and pain, honour and dishonour. He to whom a clod of earth,

86

stone and gold are the same, he has achieved the Yoga of stead-
fastness and harmony.

All philosophies of the world indicate that Man's capacity for good
is infinite. Why then is the history of the world a long story of
suffering? If we view our present century alone, the amount of
suffering to which man and beast have been subjected staggers the
imagination. Why?

Because if Man has an infinite capacity for good he also has a
capacity for evil, not an infinite capacity since evil is ultimately self-
destructive and therefore finite, but nevertheless uniquely great. I
quote here from the Jewish prayer book, 'The Service of the Heart'.

Man was made to be free; free to do good, to love, to create, and
to beautify. Free also to do evil, to hate, to destroy, and to dese-
crate. Man finds himself in the midst of a universe which is being
formed at every moment, and he too is not yet fully grown. But in
his power to create, he has been given a special gift, for a special
task; to help in his own formation.

Man is a member of a race who are like a team of mountain
climbers engaged on a perilous ascent. Each is bound to all. Each
is free to help or hinder the ascent.

Some are strong climbers. They must help the weaker, or all will
perish. For this is the law of creation; only by love can man hope
to live.

In Man's upward climb he has often stumbled. Today it seems
he may dash himself upon the rocks below.

Again we ask why. Why has Man so often stumbled? Why all this
suffering? And will there ever be an end to it?

If I have learned anything at all from the study of Yoga it is that
everything has more than one viewpoint. *Ab initio* one thinks of
suffering as evil, destructive, fearsome, but upon further reflection
one is able to argue that the effects of suffering can be bad, neutral or
good, both morally and spiritually, according to the individual's reaction to it. And that the individual has the freedom of choice is
unquestionable.

It then becomes easy enough to view suffering as a positive challenge. Think of having nothing to overcome, nothing like a goal to
achieve. We should all probably die or go insane from sheer bore-

dom! More than that, and more gravely, Man being the aggressive animal he is would be likely to inflict suffering upon himself, more even than he has to endure from natural causes.

This leads us on to question whether suffering is, after all, the positive element of existence and whether happiness is negative in character being as it is a state of freedom from suffering. Within this context one could reason that the lower animals are more fortunate than Man, being less sensitive to both pleasure and pain. Man being more sensitive to pleasure is equally more sensitive to suffering.

To carry our analysis of suffering a step further we can see that over the centuries Man has deliberately increased his various needs in order to increase his pleasures, and this intensification and pursuit of pleasure has, in this century, resolved itself into chronic anxiety over money, neurosis on a scale unparalleled in history, and chronic frustration imposed by the kind of repetitive work which has to be done in order to satisfy the artificially stimulated demand for the fruits of mass production. So is Man any happier? Is he indeed any healthier? It is a well known medical fact that many degenerative diseases are caused by Man's failure to live in harmony with his real nature. Those who understand Yoga know that even wrong thinking influences the various parts of the body, by some excess or defect of function, to the detriment of the total organism.

We know that most people spend their lives in the pursuit of a state which they call happiness but which they are scarcely able to define. Even philosophers are not wholly in agreement as to what constitutes the state of happiness, for the simple reason that all the elements appertaining to the notion of happiness are essentially empirical, that is they stem from actual experience.

Let us suppose that an individual's conception of happiness is wealth, or to put it another way, total freedom from poverty. In his pursuit of wealth he will attract envy, cares and anxiety to himself and his family. Again let us suppose that a man's notion of happiness is knowledge (or freedom from ignorance). Is it not possible that in furthering his intellectual achievements he will also become more and more aware of how little he really knows? Could this be called a state of happiness? And again supposing that a man considers that happiness means a long life. Has he any guarantee at all that this would not be one long torment? And the man who has suffered a long illness, does he not believe that happiness is a return to health? But can he be sure that he will not fall ill again, or suffer a disabling accident? And is this not a cause for further anxiety?

So, on any principle, man is unable to determine with any degree of certainty what constitutes true happiness. He can only act on empirical counsels of regimen, frugality and self-respect and so on, which in his experience have, on the whole, most promoted his well-being.

Basically the problem is that happiness is not an ideal of reason but of imagination and it seems that all roads ultimately lead Man back to a state of suffering. And so we are driven to ask ourselves again—why? Also can we possibly make our lives more tolerable and if so, how?

If we can accept that suffering is the positive, and *not* the negative element of existence, then we can regulate our expectations accordingly. So that every tranquil moment, being a bonus, is therefore precious and to be lived and enjoyed to the full, here and now. And in our inter-personal relationships, if we can accept that Man is an imperfect being we then have no right to feel hurt or surprised if the conduct of others leaves much to be desired. In other words, if we can accept what *is* instead of what we would like, or think we would like, then we can begin to acquire some of the positive virtues such as forbearance, social usefulness, and above all, kindness.

Viewed in this light it is not difficult to see that suffering is a necessary part of being alive and that if we build walls around ourselves in an effort to shut out suffering we will shut out life as well. One of the most universal sources of unhappiness is the habit of putting off living to some fictional future date. 'When we have five hundred pounds we will get married.' 'When I have a house of my own I will buy a piano and take lessons.' 'When I am earning two (or three) thousand a year I will start to do some serious reading.' We hear this sort of thing all the time. Reading it in cold print you can see just how fatal this attitude of mind is. It is called deferred living. And the trouble about this approach to life is that so often events spoil our best laid intentions and plans and if living is deferred for too long people can grow too old, too ill, too tired or too lazy to do what they originally wanted to do. Then we hear the ubiquitous 'if only'. 'If only I had learnt to paint, play the 'cello, make jewellery, grow roses.'

But 'if only' can be, and very often is, an excuse people make to themselves and others out of fear—fear of doing something imperfectly, fear of the derision of others, fear of trying and failing to reach their own imagined high standards. Or as I said, it can be plain laziness. But one way and another, over-cautious people are unhappy and must always be the losers in terms of real living. He who never makes a mistake never makes anything at all. Need I labour the point?

We could examine every possible aspect of life on this planet and find that in everything we do there is an element of suffering. It is inescapable. All we can do is accept it as a part of life and in accepting, go beyond it. When we read the Bhagavad Gita we learn that only through self-abnegation and love can we eradicate evil, folly and ignorance, those three elements of the ego which prevent us from becoming aware of the spark of divinity which illumines Man's inner Self. For those who find the word divinity unacceptable one could substitute the word majesty. Ultimately it is not the words that matter but the meaning they convey.

We live in a world of suffering, a world continuously at war because it clearly lacks the intellectual and spiritual prerequisites to the achievement of peace.

I call God long-suffering and patient precisely because He permits evil in the world. I know, too, that I shall never know God if I do not wrestle against evil, even at the cost of life itself.

MAHATMA GANDHI, 1869–1948

Chapter 6

TENSION AND ANXIETY

Better to hunt in fields, for health unbought,
Than fee the doctor for a nauseous draught.
The wise, for cure, on exercise depend;
God never made his work for man to mend.

DRYDEN

THE BRAIN is continuously receiving nervous impulses arising from three sources: environment, the body and the mind. Any information appertaining to the environment reaches us through our five physical senses: hearing, sight, smell, taste and touch. As a general rule we are aware of these sensations. But the brain also receives information from all parts of the body and we are not always consciously aware of this. As an example we manage to maintain our physical balance without being conscious most of the time that we are doing so.

A more complex system of impulses arises within the brain itself and is manifested on different levels:

1. Conscious thoughts, doubts, anxieties, feelings of like and dislike and so on.

2. Conflicts, worries, fears arising from the unconscious but which can readily be raised to the level of the conscious.

3. The unconscious itself with its memories of all our past experiences and their associated fears and hopes. These memories, although beyond recall except under certain circumstances, have a vital and continuous effect on our mental processes by reason of the impulses which arise from them.

If the number of impulses becomes too great the brain becomes unable to integrate them and we experience this state of incomplete integration as anxiety or nervous tension. Both the body and the mind react to anxiety in their particular ways. Biologically we have inherited the ancient defence mechanism of a powerful response to the threat of attack from enemies. The result is a tensing of muscles, raised blood pressure, an increased heartbeat, cold hands, prickling scalp. This outmoded bodily reaction to anxiety does not enable us to tolerate either the cause or the distress of the unpleasant sensation. Mentally, the reaction to anxiety is a pathological over-alertness of mind, the result of which is an over-sensitization to minor irritations. This causes restlessness, physical and mental, and an inability to relax but can also, when the anxiety is intense, cause apathy, an inability to concentrate, to move or to speak. This is due to a self-regulating mechanism which inhibits severe or overwhelming anxiety reactions.

It is possible, indeed fairly common, for people who have suffered from long standing anxiety to become so accustomed to it as to accept it as normal. When this stage is reached the sufferer no longer knows he is anxious. The various signs of anxiety are often elusive so it will be helpful, I think, to my readers, if I list some of the main ones.

1. physical tension
2. nervous tension
3. irritability
4. apprehension
5. insomnia
6. fatigue
7. depression
8. lack of concentration
9. difficulty in inter-personal relationships
10. restlessness
11. obsession
12. phobia
13. speech impediments
14. palpitations
15. chest pain, especially on the right side
16. indigestion
17. allergic reactions, i.e. skin rash, asthma
18. migraine and nervous headaches
19. painful menstruation.

Yoga's method of relieving tension and anxiety is based on a technique which assists the natural processes of the mind. This method is widely accepted because it is effective no matter what may be the cause of the anxiety. This is not to say that everything is plain sailing, on the contrary a high degree of co-operation is required of the Yoga student, and here we meet the problem of self-discipline. Anyone, or almost anyone, will readily accept the idea of physical exercise as a source of bodily health, and this accounts for the universal popularity of Hatha Yoga. But the very same people who will happily perform a half hour a day of Yoga postures and pranayama (breathing and breath control) sometimes have difficulty in remembering to impose upon themselves the smallest degree of mental discipline. The Yoga technique therefore has a common sense list of do's and don'ts.

1. Do not expect the graph of your recovery from anxiety to be a straight line. You will be certain to have your off days when you could easily become disheartened if not forewarned.

2. Do try not to be discouraged or impatient if your overall recovery appears to be slow.

3. Do try to cultivate the habit of mental discipline and self-control throughout the day. When the habit is established you will be able to relax your constant vigil.

4. Do try to condition yourself to enjoying this discipline.

5. Do try to remember to hold on to any feeling of mental relaxation which you may achieve for as long as you can. Try not to do anything which might disturb your mood.

6. Do try to perform *actions* in a relaxed manner. You will find yourself more efficient, both physically and mentally.

7. Do try to practise Yoga relaxation exercises regularly, preferably on rising and before retiring to bed.

The following exercises are all effective in relieving tension.

Relaxing the Face and Neck

1. *Head roll.* Sit on a hard chair, back straight, stomach held in. Close your eyes and let your head fall back without moving any other part of the body. Roll the head round clockwise six times letting it drop loosely onto the chest and backwards as far as it can go. Keeping your eyes closed roll the head anti-clockwise six times.

2. *Ear to shoulder.* Still seated, and holding the shoulders absolutely still, bend the neck to the right, trying to touch your shoulder with your right ear. Repeat to the left which completes the exercise. Perform six times.

3. *Tortoise.* Sitting straight and still push out the chin as far as possible. You will feel the pressure in your neck at the base of the skull. Perform six times.

4. *Side to side stretch.* Holding the shoulders still, turn your head as far as possible to the right, keeping your chin well off your chest. Repeat to the left. Perform six times alternately.

5. *Up and down stretch*. Keeping the seated position, and keeping your eyes closed allow your head to fall back as far as possible, allowing your mouth to open naturally. Do not lean backwards in your chair. Let the head drop forward onto the chest which completes the exercise. Perform six times.

The following exercises are performed lying down:

1. Lie on your back with a pillow under your head, keeping your eyes closed. Try to push your head back through the pillow as hard as you can while breathing normally. Hold for six seconds and then relax. Perform six times.

2. Lie on your face with your forehead on the pillow. Close your eyes and push your head down as hard as you can. Hold for six seconds. Repeat the exercise six times.

3. Lie on your right side with both hands under your right cheek. Push your head down against your hands as hard as you can. Hold for six seconds. Perform six times and then turn on your left side and repeat.

The following exercises are performed seated on a straight-backed chair.

1. Clasp your hands behind your neck with fingers interlinked. Push hands hard against your neck and at the same time push your head back as hard as you can. Hold for six seconds. Repeat six times.

2. Link your fingers together and place the palms of your hands against your forehead, with your elbows pointing straight ahead. Push your forehead forward as hard as you can and hold for six seconds. Perform six times.

3. Place the palm of your right hand against your right ear. Push your hand hard against your skull and at the same time press your head against your hand. Hold for six seconds. Perform six times, then repeat with the left hand against your left ear.

4. Yawning. Open your mouth and eyes as wide as you can. Feel the pull of every muscle in your face. Hold for four seconds. Perform six times.

5. Link your fingers together and put the palms of your hands against the back of your head. Press your hands hard against your head and your head against your hands. Hold for four seconds. Perform six times.

6. Sit up straight on your chair with your arms down by your sides. Pull both shoulders down as hard as you can, holding the position for four seconds. Perform six times.

As well as practising relaxation exercises it should be remembered that the normal way to relieve emotional pressure is not by trying to keep a 'stiff upper lip' but by letting go in the form of tears, talk-it out, or best of all, laughter. It also helps if you can turn your mind to some absorbing occupation, but this is not always possible. The practice of physical exercises is well known to have a calming effect upon the mind and in fact it is impossible to be both physically completely relaxed and emotionally tense. The opposite also applies: it is impossible to be emotionally at peace and in a state of physical tension. The mind and body interact upon each other.

Although no one can get through life without the usual ups and downs of everyday existence, it is only common sense to do one's best to avoid any kind of stress which can remain as a focus of anxiety and depression. And it should be remembered that few inter-personal relationships are without some emotional aspect, and that every emotional experience helps to build up tension. With practice the individual can learn how best to avoid a heavy build-up of tension by working off emotional pressure in socially beneficial ways.

Chapter 7

ADOLESCENCE

On his bold visage middle-age
Had slightly press'd its signet sage,
Yet had not quench'd the open truth
And fiery vehemence of youth;
Forward and frolic glee was there,
The will to do, the soul to dare.
        SIR WALTER SCOTT
        'The Lady of the Lake'

THERE must always have been some degree of misunderstanding between the adolescent and his elders, but apparently at no time in
history has the generation gap been more apparent and difficult to
negotiate than in the present day. The fact of being misunderstood
causes frustration, the manifestation of which is usually aggression.
This is commonly regarded as an inevitable characteristic of adolescence. Yet both psychologists and Yoga teachers believe that society
in general, and the parents and teachers of adolescents in particular,
must take a considerable amount of responsibility for the existence of
this problem whose causes are mainly due to a lack of understanding.

On the other hand the adolescent suffers from very real handicaps
which are intensified by the attitude of the society in which he moves.
Older people resent the absence of respect and courtesy in the present-
day adolescent, yet find it difficult to allow him a status of equality in
view of their own upbringing at a time when young people did not
enjoy the degree of freedom that they do today. The adolescent re-
acts, quite understandably, by displaying churlishness, indifference,
even rudeness. Neither can understand the other's point of view.

A condition of brooding unhappiness is all too common in the
adolescent. Although psychologists know very well that it is a by-
product of self-consciousness, few people who have not made a study
of psychology can understand the very real agony of mind suffered
by many people in the 'teen' years. It is a matter which requires

serious attention for many reasons. If subjected to too many brutal attacks from contemporaries or too great an indifference or lack of understanding from the older generation, adolescent self-consciousness can at best result in a lack of physical and mental drive and efficiency, and at worst grow into a crippling neurosis which marks the individual for life.

In order to understand this common but agonizing condition it is advisable first to stop to define terms. Self-consciousness can be defined in Yogic terms as an awareness of self as an individual, entirely separate from other individuals, or it can mean simply shyness. These two aspects of self-consciousness have at least one point of comparison in that both are accompanied by feelings of isolation and anxiety mixed with equivocal feelings of love/hate towards certain other people.

Life can be made much more tolerable for the self-conscious adolescent by a sympathetic approach from others, and in saying sympathetic I stress that I do not mean a maudlin attitude which would be intolerable to a sensitive adolescent, but mental participation in another's condition. The Yogic approach would be an attempt to see the position from the adolescent's point of view, a precept which is so often overlooked. There is no lack of desire to understand this problem in those who are in any way involved with or responsible for adolescents, but more is required if the desire to help is to be resolved into effective action. For one thing older people with years of experience behind them are often convinced that their 'superior' point of view would appeal to and be easily accepted by adolescents, a conviction which is for the most part fallacious. Many older people have an imperfect recollection of their childhood and adolescence although few are aware of the extent to which their recollections are distorted and incomplete and still fewer would readily admit to it. And so the older person has first to adjust his or her point of view to that of the adolescent before any kind of purposeful communication can be achieved.

It is vital to understand that an adolescent who is self-conscious is *emotionally isolated*. When at school he has relatively infrequent contact with his parents and but superficial contact with his teachers, thereby falling between two stools. Consequently he often suffers in silence, being unsure of who to confide his problems to, and the danger here is that he can easily withdraw so much into himself that his social sense and emotional development are inhibited to the ex-

97

tent of crippling his inter-personal relationships when he leaves school and tries to assume his place in society.

The self-conscious adolescent should not and must not be judged by *adult standards* but by the standards which apply to youth in general and the individual adolescent in particular. Of course the shy adolescent is evasive, of course he is often inarticulate, of course he is often difficult. These are difficult years for any sensitive human being. But except in extreme cases the confusion of the adolescent is intermittent, and mercifully the sheer business of living brings with it increased self-confidence and a feeling of being a worthwhile member of society.

In the meantime what can be done to reach the mind and understand the feelings of the adolescent who suffers from these problems? Is there a yardstick of comparison which will enable us to take effective steps to mitigate them? Self-consciousness has as many causes as there are individuals but the following are perhaps the most important. A very common focus of acute shyness or self-consciousness is some imperfect, unusual or disliked physical characteristic, i.e. underweight, overweight, tallness, shortness, skin blemishes, bright red or carroty hair (especially in a boy), large hands, a stammer, excessively large feet, and of course actual deformity. While there is no standard by which to evaluate these despised physical characteristics, the determining factor is almost always the comments or jeers of others. Youth is by no means all sweetness and light: young people can be brutal to each other.

Dress is important to the adolescent, and older people should allow him a free hand in the choosing of his own clothes even if they do not meet with the approval of his elders. So long as the adolescent feels comfortable (and anonymous) in them it is best to leave well alone. To dress in a manner likely to set him apart from his fellows would be intolerable. The main thing is that if the adolescent chooses to dress in what appears to be a bizarre or slovenly manner it is no kindness to force him to have his clothes made in Savile Row!

Sport is as important as dress to the adolescent. Outstanding ability at outdoor games is a certain passport to popularity while even moderate ability ensures that one is at least accepted. It is futile to try to reason with a teenager who is academically bright but who cannot score a goal or bang a ball over a net. Adolescence is a time when values are judged by peculiar standards and priorities seem to be the result of irrational thought. But older people should beware of passing judgement from their own standpoint. The understanding of young people requires above all an adjustment of thinking, a shifting of one's point of view to that of the adolescent as I have reiterated several times in order to stress how vital this is. If therefore the adolescent undervalues his academic achievements and longs only to emulate the current tennis or football star, it is best to go along with this until such time as he is ready to understand and accept the solid worthwhile importance of a high intelligence.

Shyness is almost the hall-mark of the adolescent, and although agonizing to the individual is often very appealing to others, especially older people to whom an over-confident teenager is vaguely disquieting. Shyness parades in many guises and some of them such as bad manners, toughness, and arrogance are very difficult to live with. Although trying in the extreme to older people it should always be remembered that these are the adolescent's *defences* against what to him appears to be a hostile world.

The shy adolescent will go to absurd lengths to avoid emotional situations, largely because he fears his own emotions and his inability to control them. Those who are shy and sensitive will protect their sensitivity at all costs even to the extent of appearing morose, uncooperative and aggressive. And of course aggression is another hall-mark of adolescence. This shows itself in word and deed and is in fact a very effective means of self-protection. Teenagers are notorious for discovering and attacking the well-guarded secrets of their contemporaries and possibly the only defence against this is a retreat behind a thorny exterior. And as his armour must have no chinks in it the adolescent cannot afford to relax his vigil for a moment even when in the company of, and sometimes *particularly* when in the company of, his own family and close friends.

His attitude towards any kind of authority is almost deliberately recalcitrant and older people would do well to remember that adolescence is rather like the spring which is a period of intense growth and movement. The movement is inevitably *away* from adult standards and towards his own, and the adult will find that he can no longer compel the adolescent to think and behave as he (the adult) thinks fit and proper. One cause of tension between the parent generation and the adolescent is the former's anxiety about the adolescent's health and well-being. Leaving aside those parents who clutch at the matter of health as their final hold over their children, the adolescent is still almost unbearably irritated by what he terms nagging about health 'for his own good'.

So how does one steer a safe course on this matter? There is no easy answer as much depends upon the individuals concerned, but the following points will serve as a general guide.

1. At all costs avoid direct inteference.

2. The older person's approach should always be determined by the reactions of the individual adolescent concerned.

3. Any points of particular anxiety to older people concerning the adolescent's health and personal hygiene, e.g. the brushing of teeth, smoking, drinking, posture, regular meals, bathing and sleep can seldom be introduced into a conversation without boring and antagonizing the adolescent. It requires so much subtlety that it is beyond any normal adult, and in any case it doesn't usually have the slightest effect.

4. In the absence of any choice one way or another the adult is advised to leave well alone concerning health matters when the issue is a fairly trivial one. In matters of real ill health the adolescent will be likely to exercise common sense and a doctor should be able to do the rest, or if the adolescent displays any interest in Yoga the Yoga teacher usually has a great deal of influence, even with adolescents!

5. One of the main causes of child/parent conflict is the desire of adolescents to become fully adult and the equally strong desire of many parents to keep them children. The adolescent has a natural reaction again pressure, common sense restrictions, indeed any form of authority at all, because it suggests that he is still being treated as a child. On the other hand the parent fears for the safety of his offspring in an adult world. This fear has various aspects: there is the fear that the recklessness of the adolescent will lead him into serious trouble, the fear that his indiscretion or rude behaviour will reflect on his upbringing and bring unhappiness or disgrace upon his family who were responsible for it. The fear can also be a projection of the adult's own fears. The common sense attitude to this conflict is acceptance by the adult of the younger person's point of view even when this seems unreasonable. If the adolescent is allowed to differ from his elders the game of 'getting at the old folk' will eventually pall and the adolescent will then be likely to adopt a more moderate attitude and even credit his parents and teachers with a little intelligence!

6. The difficult adolescent has a dichotomous attitude towards his

independence which may be quite unknown to the adult, who finds his child's behaviour incomprehensible. The fact is that the adolescent, at one and the same time, longs for freedom and independence and on the other hand fears the unknown, fears premature responsibility, and most of all fears the withdrawal of adult protection. It is vital that the adult should try to understand and accept this dichotomy.

7. The adolescent often displays bravado, and adults would do well to realize that fear often lies behind this. While he needs to feel his own strength and freedom, there is a very real fear of failure or of falling short. And because of his need for self-respect the adolescent will be reluctant to shirk any kind of new experience and will often rush to meet it out of sheer defiance.

8. As a general rule the adolescent will be reluctant to take advice concerning any aspect of behaviour from parents, guardians or teachers for the simple reason that it is these very people who have controlled his conduct for so many years. The adult will avoid a great deal of unpleasantness if he bears this in mind.

9. Adolescents have a fierce desire for privacy of possession and will hoard apparently useless trifles. If the adult should even attempt to tidy up or the adolescent suspects him of prying there is a risk of a serious breach in the relationship. The needs of the adolescent should be respected until this phase has passed.

10. Another source of conflict is the adult's suspicion of any outside forces which may impinge on the adolescent. If the adult displays the slightest annoyance the reaction of the adolescent will be defiance. The only common sense answer is to offer hospitality to each and every new friend the adolescent may wish to bring home, no matter how undesirable they may be, and on no account to criticize. The adolescent will usually be sensible enough to measure his new friends against his familiar background and discard those whom he finds wanting.

11. The adult is naturally hurt and perplexed when the child who used to confide everything to him gradually turns into a reticent, even secretive adolescent. However this is apparently a normal phenomenon reflecting the ever-present need for independence and as such should be respected.

12. Adolescents are notoriously moody and it should be pointed out that moods are as much a reflection of inner needs as of external circumstances and that these constantly react upon each other. The

needs of the adolescent have increased yet circumstances often preclude their being satisfied. The desire for independence, for instance, is one basic need which obviously cannot be fulfilled until the adolescent leaves school and earns enough to live away from home. Even then he may continue for some years to be emotionally dependent upon his elders.

13. During the rather trying phase of adolescence the affection of the parent will be severely tried at many points. He will need a considerable amount of tact and patience, which is good mind-training for the adult. And although he has little choice in the matter he will ultimately find it rewarding to the relationship if he learns to treat the adolescent as an equal and learns to recognize that the younger person has a right to his own point of view, and also has the right to relapse (as he sometimes will) from adult standards. Fortunately most parents have a natural sympathy for their offspring, but this does not imply either the need for sentimentality in dealing with the adolescent or relieving him from making any effort. A middle course is best, and at all times it is wise to let the adolescent live his own life, and make his own mistakes, because too much interference can cause resentment and prevent the younger person from finding his own feet. I often hear tales of conflict from those of my pupils who have adolescent children and from my adolescent pupils themselves. Adolescents who choose to study Yoga are at a distinct advantage because they are directed by the teacher how to discover and accept their real selves, but even then there can be a slipping back from growing self-confidence because of pressures at home. The parent does not understand and often imposes his ideas (unacceptable to the younger person) and even his will upon a mind which is growing and searching for an identity.

To parent and offspring, Yoga has this to say. Any person, if he is to evolve successfully towards maturity and independence and realize his own innate potential, must find his way alone, although at the same time he may not want to sever contact with his parents. They on their part must show wisdom in observing from a distance and sometimes (but only sometimes) pointing out what they consider is the way. At the same time the adolescent has a right (which he will often exercise) to choose another way. It may not be the best way for him but he will learn from his mistake. And when he does reach emotional maturity, a stage which occurs long after intellectual maturity is reached, he will be certain to see the world in a focus entirely different from that of his elders.

14. The younger person often feels afraid and uncertain along the difficult climb to adulthood although he would not care to admit it, and the adult can rest assured that in many ways (more ways than he perhaps imagines) his love, moral support and his company are needed as much at this time as at any other time in his child's life. The adolescent is reminded that it is not an easy time for the parent who is vulnerable where his child is concerned and can easily be hurt or become agitated when the offspring behaves too recklessly. It is possible to display a little consideration without losing one's individuality.

15. A point in mind-training in all forms of Yoga, and one which particularly applies to the problems of adolescence, is the matter of taking the consequences of one's own actions. The adult need not and should not hide from the adolescent the results of his (the adolescent's) actions but at the same time a long-suffering or disapproving attitude is to be avoided. Adolescents tend to label adults and categorize them and they are very sensitive to people who approve and disapprove of them. Other categories are those who are sympathetic and those who are not, those who are easily angered or irritated and those who are not, those who understand and those who do not. To the child the parents were gods who filled the horizon; they are no longer so to the adolescent who has developed the faculty of objectivity regarding his elders. And more than one adolescent has learned to despise one or both of his parents, one or more of his teachers. This is often due to a failure of understanding on both sides. To the older person the adolescent's behaviour and viewpoint are so bewildering that he takes refuge behind an attitude of disapproval. The adolescent on the other hand despises the older person for not being clever enough to understand him.

The adolescent is bewildered by the physiological and emotional changes within himself and is handicapped by his bewilderment. He can be helped only by a tolerance born of wisdom and the business of living itself, and by love and humour, the latter more important than some adults believe. Adolescence is not a tragedy: it is a natural process of growth.

Chapter 8

THE OUTSIDER

I see crowds of people walking around in a ring.
T. S. ELIOT *The Waste Land* (1922)

THE OUTSIDER is the title of a famous novel by the French Nobel prize winner, Albert Camus, and it is also the title of an examination of the various aspects of the Outsider temperament by Colin Wilson (1956). But long before Camus Outsiders had been the subject of literature even though they were not known by this term. Schopenhauer, having read the Upanishads, adopted the term Maya, meaning illusion, and used it to illustrate his contention that the world we see around us is mere illusion obscuring reality. This point of view is held by the majority of Outsiders.

But it is one thing to quote from the Gita and the Upanishads about Maya or illusion, and from other books in which the Outsider is portrayed, and quite another to feel oneself to be an Outsider. For instance, when I ask a new pupil, 'Why do you want Yoga?' the answer I get is often, 'I don't know' or, 'I seem to be missing something.' These are people who have embarked upon a search—a search for answers, for an identity, for some kind of justification for their being in a way 'different' from other people. Seldom do they know what they are searching for, except in a vague sense; they only know that their life is, and always has been, a kind of quest, and that they seem to be out of step with the rest of humanity. But not entirely, because even though these people are Outsiders, if two of them happen to meet they often form close and enduring relationships. For if they are not on the same wavelength as the rest of humanity, at least Outsiders speak the same language. Because these are thinking people, people who have dismissed all pretence and all that is super-ficial in life, and who look for underlying truths in every facet of their lives.

But first, in writing of the Outsider it is necessary to define exactly what the term implies. Let us say he is a being apart, a person who is one degree nearer to Reality than his fellows, or to use the words of Henri Barbusse in his novel, *L'Enfer*, one who 'sees too deep and too much'.

The Outsider has been beloved of writers from William Blake to the present day. Many of the world's greatest men of letters have made the Outsider the subject of their works, among them Tolstoy, Dostoievsky, James Joyce, Hemingway, T. S. Eliot, Franz Kafka, W. B. Yeats, Nietzsche, Thomas Traherne, Shaw, Hulme, and Sartre. But what, we may ask, is the fascination of the Outsider so far as writers are concerned, what characterizes him and what makes him different from his fellows? One could, I believe, sum it up in just four words 'a sense of unreality'. Or to put it another way, he does not feel at ease in the world.

But the Outsider is not merely a figment of literature, and we therefore cannot read about and then dismiss him as having nothing to do with us and the substantial world in which we live. It would be so much more comfortable if we could! For better or worse some of us *are* Outsiders, or someone close to us could be one, and so the Outsider's particular problems are very real, they have to be lived through, in many cases suffered through.

The most urgent of these problems is the 'know thyself' one. The Outsider has a compulsive need to achieve the maximum expression of self, if possible in some imaginative form.

The Outsider has a strong case against our social order and lives his life in a kind of moral anarchy according to the laws of his own nature. He is almost always an introvert, is often but not always artistically gifted, and is usually misunderstood, to a greater or lesser degree, except by other Outsiders. He (or she) is further characterized by an inability to feel at ease in the insulated world of the bourgeois, unable as he is to ignore that which the comfortable bourgeois is quite able and content to ignore, namely the chaotic state of life beneath the bland conventions of society.

The Outsider thinks too much, sees too much, feels too much. He is abnormally sensitive to world suffering, and even when financially stable himself, cannot ignore the poverty and deprivation of others. So if the term Outsider seems, superficially at least, alarming, it does have underlying connotations of artistic ability, a strong humanitarianism, and a high degree of intelligence. In many ways it is a privilege to have an Outsider temperament, although it has its price, as we shall see.

The Yogic attitude towards the Outsider is one of acceptance, and the injunction to every student is to accept that there is no way of avoiding the issue—if you are an Outsider you can never live successfully as an 'Insider', and vice versa, and it is both futile and cowardly to dwell on the 'might have been'.

Basically we have a choice of three attitudes towards life and what we are: that of the vegetable, that of the aggressive competitor, and that of the giver. The human vegetable lives, calm and complacent, at the lowest intellectual level consistent with humanity. He thinks only as much as is necessary to stay alive. The aggressive competitor conducts his life in the spirit of 'what can I get out of it'. Such an attitude has its positive aspect and also a negative one. On the one hand it has been responsible for the great discoveries throughout history, and on the other it lies behind dictatorship, exploitation, war, and the disintegration of inter-personal relationships. The attitude of the giver implies a recognition of the relationship of the individual to his fellow men. It is essentially an attitude of human co-operation.

The Outsider can be found on all three levels of existence. Those who are both human vegetables and Outsiders are usually neurotic, that is to say they have some personality and/or emotional imbalance. Outsiders on the other two levels are engaged upon a search for a significant aim in life. Having once obtained a glimpse of better things, better that is on an intellectual and spiritual plane, although the purely material plane can be of equal importance to many Outsiders, they can never again be content with the superficial or the humdrum. And because life cannot be lived on a continual high peak of drama and excitement, the Outsider often goes through life in a state of unease, unable to accept that human existence has its crests and troughs and unwilling to make compromises with his own difficult nature.

Outsiders are rare beings, pandas in a world of sheep, and often they are unhappy at being different until chance meetings with other Outsiders give them an opportunity to communicate. It is then that they come to realize that it is neither a good nor a bad thing to be an Outsider—it is simply one way to be. But it is essential if you are an Outsider to recognize the fact and adjust your behaviour-pattern to reflect your real nature. Unfortunately all is not plain sailing—parents bring up their children to be like themselves and if one or more of the children happen to have the Outsider temperament it could take years for the child to discover his or her real nature. Life can be, and very often is, interesting to the Outsider, but easy it never is, especially in childhood and adolescence.

The Outsider's world is essentially a dichotomy: on the one hand there is the world of order and social convention in which he is required to make the right noises (or finds it expedient to do so voluntarily). On the other hand there is his own private anarchic world. If the Outsider tries to accept the concept of the former world he will one day wake up to the realization of his own moral cowardice. If he accepts only his own inner world he will be isolated from his fellow beings. This is one of the Outsider's dilemmas. Another one is that he is usually good human material but lacking a goal towards which to aim his life-effort, and is therefore constantly in danger of degenerating into neurosis, through either idleness or lack of physical and mental exercise. These are the pathetic Outsiders who live a kind of twilight existence on the edge of society, belonging nowhere.

Yet another danger is the evasion of work for which the neurotic Outsider will have or invent a variety of excuses. The most common of these is that he has not found the 'right' occupation for his abilities. Having tried in a half-hearted manner any number of occupations he is then armed with these tangible attempts to find satisfactory work and can safely retire with a clear conscience into the world of the idle, having proved there is no kind of work for him in the world. Unfortunately (and the Outsider well knows this), there is no room for self-respect if he chooses to live this way.

And yet many Outsiders live under the constant threat of neurosis. Every age has its plagues, and neurosis is the plague of the jet age. It is not a disease but a fallacious life-technique characterized by various attempts to escape from life and to evade mature social responsibilities. The neurosis is based upon a lack of understanding of the common sense laws of human behaviour and from this is born fear and anxiety. If we examine the ten cardinal characteristics of the neurosis it will easily be seen why Outsiders are particularly vulnerable to it.

1. Lack of knowledge of what social co-operation is about.
2. The primacy of the subject's ego and the cultivation of same to the point of uniqueness.
3. An undercurrent of fear and anxiety.
4. The emotional establishment of a *subjective* feeling of power, superiority and security.

5. The aiming at a false (neurotic) goal.
6. Refusal to co-operate when help is offered. The refusal often takes the form of a denial that help is needed.
7. Some form of scapegoat is necessary.
8. A refusal to be responsible for one's own actions, especially when failure is the result.
9. A sense of futility.
10. Emotional isolation.

The ten points above add up to moral cowardice, an unwillingness to be subjected to the day-to-day tests of ordinary life. A neurotic Outsider will go to absurd lengths to fill up his day with important-sounding activities. He is always seemingly in a great hurry, rushing from one thing to another but never able to specify just why everything is so urgent. He lives in a useless world of make-believe. In fact 'useless' is the key-word in any discussion of neurosis, a mind-state which can be very useful to the subject but is not of the slightest use to the rest of mankind.

But the Outsider is by no means necessarily neurotic although the state of being neurotic would *tend* to make the subject an Outsider type.

The neurotic and the Outsider have at least one thing in common: they are isolated from their fellow men, from their joys and sorrows, and of course their problems. Instead they have a whole set of problems of their own. Further, the sphere of their activity is restricted to the smallest radius consonant with being human.

A rare and unique type of Outsider is the visionary, the person of outstanding intellectual and/or spiritual brilliance. This Outsider is supremely beneficial to mankind, an example in Yoga being Sri Ramakrishna. A singular background helped to mould his character. His formative years, spent in a small village in Bengal, were idyllic, and from the first he displayed great spirituality. As he grew older it became apparent that he was able to live on a plane of almost continuous intensity by means of an extraordinary inner harmony which he attained by contemplation.

From childhood he sought his own company and he worked ceaselessly to achieve complete detachment from the world. He was a spiritual giant, indeed a saint, and in every way an Outsider. His knowledge of life can be summed up in the following words from the Gita, Chapter 11:

The unreal never is. The Real never is not.
Men possessed of the knowledge of the Truth fully know these things.

Chapter 9

THE VALUE OF SILENCE

'Silentio et tenebris animus alitur'
The mind is nourished by darkness and silence.
PLINY THE YOUNGER

WE LIVE in the Age of Noise and because we are conditioned to it from birth, especially if we grow up in the big cities, we hardly notice the din that assaults our senses from morning until night.

Technologically the achievements of this century stagger the imagination but society has paid a heavy price by way of an incalculable increase in the physical stress ailments: ulcers, migraine, heart disease, high blood pressure to name but a few, and psychologically we see the results of the damage in almost universal nervous tension, in insomnia, in neuroses, in fact in every conceivable mental and emotional disorder. Psychiatrists are grossly overworked, psychiatric clinics are full to bursting point, and mental hospitals have long waiting lists.

We can lay blame for all this havoc wherever our peace is most ferociously shattered. If you live near an airport you can blame the noise of aircraft. If you travel to work by train or underground your heads are filled with nerve-shattering noise. Television is by no means blameless, but worse than its noise, because more intrusive, is its advertising which creates unrest, desire, and dissatisfaction with what one has. Advertising has its value to society in bringing to the public notice that which is available on the market, but it can be, and often is, wholly destructive to one's peace of mind.

And so at no time in history has Yoga been more necessary. It provides an antidote to all this century's distracting and stress-making activity. The value of silence is all over the Bhagavad Gita, the Vedas, the Upanishads and indeed all India's great books. But the great thinkers of other countries, too, have expressed their ideas about silence, some in poetry, some in incomparable prose, but all reiterating what is to be found in the works of Yoga's great sages. And so in devoting the rest of this chapter to the illustration of this with quotations, I hope to impress upon my readers the universality of Yogic thought and perhaps remind them of some of the World's great books which, in the stress of modern life, they have forgotten, overlooked, or perhaps have yet to enjoy.

Silence is the Mother of Truth.

DISRAELI

Silence does not make mistakes.

Hindu proverb

The tree of silence bears the fruit of peace.

Arab proverb

In quietness and in confidence shall be your strength.

ISAIAH

He that moves in the world of the senses and yet keeps those senses in complete harmony finds rest in quietness. And in this quietness sorrow is destroyed, for when the heart has found tranquility, wisdom has also found peace.

The Bhagavad Gita, II

The Yogi should constantly practise the harmony of soul; in a secret place, retiring into deepest solitude, alone, with the mind and the body subdued, and free from desire for possessions. Let him sit in a place that is restful and pure, with Kusha grass and above that a tiger or deer skin.
Let him rest there on that seat and practise Yoga for the purification of the heart, with body and mind in peace, his soul in silence before Me [Krishna].

The Bhagavad Gita

The Self in man has four conditions.
The first is the conscious life which enjoys the seven outer gross elements.
The second is the inner life of dreams, which enjoys the seven subtle inner elements in its own silence and solitude.
The third is dreamless sleep, the life of silent consciousness.

The fourth is Atman (the Self) in its own pure state, the life of a wakened super-consciousness, beyond thought and ineffable.

The Mandukya Upanishad

He who knows speaks not.
He who speaks knows not.
Close thou the gates and doors
Soften the brilliant lights
Turn noise into silence
and behold
The wonder of Oneness.

The Tao Te Ching, LVI

Translated by Juan Mascaró

Better than a thousand useless words is a single word that gives peace.

The Dhammapada

Having been shown the path of Yoga, and having listened to the speech of Lord Krishna, of supreme glory, Uddhava's eyes filled with tears and his voice was choked with emotion and he was silent. He could utter nothing and stood with folded hands.

The Last Message of Sri Krishna

Use the repetition of the word OM to silence the mind and deflect all distraction and negative emotion.

Patanjali's Yoga

No speech ever uttered or utterable is worth comparison with silence.

THOMAS CARLYLE

Nam nulli tacuisse nocet, nocet esse locutum—For it is harmful to no one to have been silent, but it is harmful to have spoken.

CATO

Let our silent meditation be on the glorious light of Savitri. May this light illumine our minds.

Rig Veda

There is a Spirit that is mind and life, light and truth and vast spaces. He contains all works and desires and all perfumes and all tastes. He enfolds the whole universe, and in silence is loving to all.

The Chandogya Upanishad
Translated by Juan Mascaró

Adam, while he spak not, had paradys at wylle.

LANGLAND

Be silent always when you doubt your sense.

POPE

Be able to be alone. Lose not the advantage of solitude and the society of thyself, nor be only content, but delight to be alone and silent with Omniprescency. He who is thus prepared, the day is not uneasy nor the night black unto him. Darkness may bound his eyes, not his imagination. In his bed he may lie and speculate the universe, and enjoy the whole world in the hermitage of himself.

SIR THOMAS BROWNE

And the work of righteousness shall be peace; and the effect of righteous tranquility and assurance forever.

ISAIAH

The first virtu, sone, if thou wolt lere (learn)
Is to restreyne and kepe wel thy tongue.

CHAUCER

The Universe is very beautiful, yet it says nothing. The four seasons abide by a fixed law, yet they are not heard. All creation is based upon absolute principles, yet nothing speaks.
And the true Sage, taking his stand upon the beauty of the Universe, pierces the principles of things created, and thus the saying that the wise and perfect man does nothing but gaze at the Universe.

CHUANG TZU, XXII
Translated by H. A. Giles

As a lamp in a place sheltered from the wind does not flicker—

even such has been the simile used for a Yogi of tranquil mind, silently concentrating on the Self.

The Bhagavad Gita, VI

If the crow could have fed in silence, it would have had more of a feast, and much less strife and envy.

HORACE

Silence is wisdom, but the man who practises it is seldom seen.

Arabic proverb

Speech is of time, silence is of eternity.

THOMAS CARLYLE

Day after day, O Lord, shall I stand before thee face to face? With folded hands, O Lord of all worlds, shall I stand before thee face to face?
Under thy great sky in solitude and silence, with humble heart shall I stand before thee face to face?
In this laborious world of thine, tumultuous with toil and with struggle, among hurrying crowds shall I stand before thee face to face?
And when my work shall be done in this world, O Lord, alone and silent shall I stand before thee face to face?

RABINDRANATH TAGORE

Chapter 10

KARMA YOGA

Blessed is he who has found his work;
let him ask no other blessedness.

THOMAS CARLYLE
Past and Present,
Book 3 Chapter II

I AM aware that many people know of this Yoga by name only, as it is little known and seldom written about outside India. But I am convinced that it is the Yoga most relevant to the 1970s because it deals with action.

Before we examine how this Yoga is practised it is necessary for me to expose another fallacy. Many people think the word Karma means fate. It does not. The word is derived from the Sanskrit Kri which means 'to do'. Everything that we do, all action is Karma. And the word also means the effects of action. Karma in other words is work and Karma Yoga is the Yoga of Selfless work.

No Yoga is easy and it may be that Karma Yoga is so little known in the Western world because it is, in many ways, so difficult to perform properly. Yet it remains, in my opinion, the most fascinating, even though when examined in depth it becomes clear that it demands of those who practise it qualities of character given to, or attained by, comparatively few people. If we think that the goal of mankind is knowledge, and that in order to attain the highest knowledge we have to climb a mountain up which there are four main paths, we could, with impunity, regard Karma Yoga as its most formidable face. It is a challenge. Some people thrive on challenges and, having overcome them, have a greater sense of achievement than those who opted for the easier way.

To practise Karma Yoga we have to live in the world. With other Yogas one can be shut away in a room by oneself and study or concentrate or meditate in peace and silence. Not so with Karma Yoga. To practise it you need other people, you need to go out and perform your Selfless Actions in the midst of the bustle and noise of the 1970s.

All action being the display of human thought, it is the manifestation of Man's will. It follows then that as we are responsible, by all our past actions, for what we are at present, we have within us the power to make ourselves whatever we wish to be. So our characters being the sum total of all our past actions (and reactions to given situations), we may conclude that our future actions will inevitably determine what sort of person we shall become.

If we choose the way of Karma Yoga to mould our character, gain Self-Awareness, and find our way to the top of the mountain of Yoga, we must be careful, *at all times*, to direct our actions towards this goal and perform no deed, utter no word, allow no thought to cross our minds which will not carry us a step upwards. A behaviour pattern such as this requires a formidable degree of awareness of one's own character, absolute truth with oneself (which can be a harrowing experience!) and the self control which the constant practice of Yoga demands and which, in the adept, comes as second nature.

Good and evil both have a share in moulding the character, though often Man is seen at his most noble in his struggle with, and triumph over, adversity. The effect of Karma or action on character is the greatest power Man has to deal with in this aspect of Yoga. Our starting point must be the realization, the absolute acceptance, of the fact that we, and we alone, are responsible for what we are. It matters not that outside influences press in upon us from birth onwards. What is significant, and psychologically sound, is that it is our manner of dealing with situations which makes us what we are. One can therefore call Karma Yoga the 'Yoga of Cause and Effect'.

The Bhagavad Gita on the subject of Karma Yoga says explicitly that knowledge is inherent in Man, that his mind is a power-house of infinite knowledge. And that the goal of mankind is the *uncovering* of this knowledge. I refer my readers to Plato's dialogue *Meno* in which the great Greek philosopher expresses the same view.

The following example of Karma Yoga comes from the Bhagavad Gita. Arjuna, the warrior prince, is overcome with grief to discover that those he is required to kill in battle are his own kinsmen. In his perplexity he calls upon the God Vishnu, in his human form of Krishna, to advise him as to the best course of action.

Arjuna:

With my nature overpowered by grief, with my mind in confusion

116

about my duty, I supplicate Thee. Say decidedly what is for the best. I am thy disciple. Instruct me who have taken refuge in Thee.

Krishna replies at length, ending with the words:

Of that which is born death is certain; of that which is dead birth is certain. Over the unavoidable, therefore, thou oughtest not to grieve.

This last sentence means that as one cannot control the inevitable (as Arjuna cannot preserve the bodies of his kinsmen), one must work out one's own Karma (actions) according to the law of one's own being.

In reply to Arjuna's question about duty Krishna replies:

Looking at thine own Dharma [religious duty] also, thou oughtest not to waver, for there is nothing higher for a Kshatriya [a member of the warrior caste] than a righteous war.

So again Krishna enjoins Arjuna to perform action according to his own nature. This is Karma Yoga in action. And Krishna warns Arjuna:

But if thou refusest to engage in this righteous warfare, then forfeiting thine own Dharma and honour, thou shalt incur sin.

Further on Krishna tells Arjuna to grieve no more but arise and do what his religious duty requires of him, to fight. Krishna:

The wisdom of Self-realization has been declared unto thee. Hearken thou now to the wisdom of Yoga, endued with which thou shalt break through the bonds of Karma.

The meaning of this speech of Krishna's is as follows:
The Yoga referred to is Karma Yoga or that behaviour pattern which involves the working out of past actions, non-accumulation of new ones, and the working towards Self-realization with the whole of one's will. Karma Yoga is therefore self-discipline of the highest order and all actions should be directed towards this end. Anything

unworthy is to be discarded. The 'bonds of Karma' refers to the desire for results which is the effect of most actions performed by ordinary human beings. Karma Yoga is concerned with action devoid of the desire for results. This action becomes a form of worship and as such leads to awareness of the highest Self.

Positive action, selfless work, is one way of releasing the power of the human mind. Those who practise Karma Yoga must accept the fact that, in the beginning, when we examine the motivation behind the majority of our actions, we discover the extent of our selfishness. Such a discovery is a shattering experience, a blow to our self-esteem, but once the ego has recovered from the shock, knowing the exact measure of the obstacle we can then set about taking positive steps to overcome it.

The student of Karma Yoga must learn, day by day, to become less selfish. Slowly, and making a hundred mistakes on the way, and slipping back many times, he will beat a path upwards. With each upward step the way becomes easier. With each step he will realize more fully the value of selfless thought and action. As I said, Karma Yoga is not easy but there is a word to remember which will make the way less difficult.

The word is love. Every thought or action performed with love carries with it a reverberation of peace and joy. In the words of Shakespeare:

It is twice blessed, it blesseth him that gives and him that takes.

I hasten to add, for the benefit of Shakespeare devotees, that Portia of *The Merchant of Venice* was here referring to the quality of mercy, but what then is mercy if not an act of love in one of its highest forms?

It is easy to love those who are lovable to us, but to love those who are not is an achievement over one's baser nature. Some people, especially those who have harmed us, or harmed someone we love, are so repugnant to us as to be virtually impossible to love or even like. How then would a follower of Karma Yoga deal with a situation such as this? It has been set down in the Gita in no uncertain terms what he should, and should not do regarding these alien beings. He should never commit any act which is harmful to another living being under any circumstances.

Krishna:

He whose mind is not shaken by adversity, who has become free from affection, fear, and wrath, is indeed a man of steady wisdom.

And further on Krishna says:

Attachment and aversion of the senses for their respective objects are natural; let none come under their sway; they are his foes.

The Gita explains this last sentence as follows: though some people are completely under the sway of their natural dispositions so that restraint is of no avail to them, the follower of Yoga should never follow their example but should strive to overcome both likes and dislikes so that all people are the same to him. He should strive to overcome the weaknesses in his own nature.

In other words we must try to love our enemies. This must be one of the most difficult things for an ordinary feeling person to do. It will, I think, be helpful here if I set down some of the less obvious interpretations of the word love.

As I have already pointed out, mercy is one of the highest manifestations of love; and this because it is almost always directed either towards our enemies or towards complete strangers, the latter, for instance, in the matter of judges passing sentence. The question of mercy, therefore, is hardly applicable in the case of those whom we love. It follows then that an act of mercy is an act of selfless love, beneficial in the first instance to the receiver, but ultimately to the bestower also in its reverberations in the form of Karma.

Compassion is another form of love, as is understanding; and there is also charity. But let me pause here to discuss this much-abused word, for many actions of a low order are committed in the name of charity. In the practise of Karma Yoga the student must appreciate that no action is worthy of the name charity unless it is performed in an attitude of complete selflessness. It is not an act of charity to give large sums of money to support worthy causes if the doner allows the fact to be published, or even repeated verbally among a handful of people. True charity is performed in secrecy and with no desire for, or expectation of, thanks from the receiver. Indeed Karma Yoga goes a step further in describing the truly charitable man as one who regards as a great *privilege* each and every opportunity of helping a fellow human being.

But having discussed the nature of true charity one cannot dismiss as worthless any act which directly or indirectly benefits another human being. People do 'good deeds' for a variety of reasons: loneliness probably comes first, but they also 'do good' in order to achieve some measure of superiority or popularity, or for the sake of their own self-esteem. Some people even perform these so-called good deeds because it is part of their social convention to do so, and not to do so would constitute a failure to conform. However a good deed is a good deed, whatever the motivation, provided someone benefits from it, but within the strict doctrines of Karma Yoga one should beware of labelling anything charity which is not an act of pure selflessness. Swami Vivekananda used to put it quite simply by saying, 'If you want to do a good work, do not trouble to think what the result will be.'

These words are applicable not only to Karma Yoga but to all the Yogas, and again the four great Yogas converge in the concept that the goal of mankind is Knowledge. The Bhagavad Gita has much to say on this subject.

Krishna:

Freed from attachment, fear and anger, absorbed in Me, taking refuge in Me, purified by the fire of knowledge, many have attained My Being.

Also:

Know that, by prostrating thyself, by questions and by service [Karma Yoga], the wise ones, those who have realized the Truth, will instruct thee in that knowledge.

Krishna speaks again to Arjuna on the subject of Knowledge:

Verily there exists nothing in this world as purifying as Knowledge. In good time, having reached perfection in Yoga, one realizes the Self.

Chapter Four of the Gita ends with Krishna's command to Arjuna:

Therefore, cutting with the sword of knowledge, this doubt about the Self, born of ignorance, residing in thy heart, take refuge in Yoga. Arise, Arjuna, arise!

The state of ignorance is discussed repeatedly in the Gita. Krishna:

> The ignorant, the man without Shraddha [one who has no faith in the words and teachings of his Guru], the doubting self, goes to destruction. The doubting self has neither this world, nor the text, nor happiness.

Krishna speaks further of universal ignorance and tells Arjuna,

> The Omnipresent takes note of the merit or demerit of none. Knowledge is enveloped in ignorance, thus do beings become deluded . . . But those whose ignorance is destroyed by the knowledge of Self—that knowledge of theirs, like the sun, reveals the Supreme Brahman.

So let us recapitulate. To practise Karma Yoga one must strive to uncover the Knowledge inherent in each and every one of us. One must accept the inevitable and work out one's own Karma (actions) according to the law of one's own being. One must practise self-discipline and perform actions with no desire for results or rewards. One must learn selflessness, and one must learn not to discriminate between likes and dislikes. At all times one should try to love and to perform actions with love. One must learn the nature of true charity, and one must endeavour to rid oneself of ignorance, the cause of all the world's evil.

Here again the four great Yogas converge in the concept that the highest ideal is complete self-abnegation, where there is no 'I' and all is 'Thou'. By exercising the power of love, in all its definitions, whenever an opportunity presents itself, the character becomes ennobled. Continuous acts of selfless love will produce their Karma. Do not look for results, but perform whatever has to be done without selfish thoughts.

To realize the Self through Karma Yoga one must rigorously and incessantly deny one's lower self. As all actions produce their Karma, continuous acts and thoughts of a base nature must inevitably produce a character of a low order. If someone strikes us, or harms us physically or verbally, it almost instinctive to strike back, if only in self-defence or self-justification. But this is the lower self in action. It takes a character of a higher order to return evil with gentleness; which brings me to another great universal concept embedded in

Yogic thought—that there is no evil which purity and gentleness cannot conquer. If one is a serious student of Yogic philosophy, if one looks beyond the printed word, the spoken thought, one must see that all Yogic concepts are universal. There is not one single Yogic principle which cannot be illustrated with words of wisdom from great thinkers, no matter what their beliefs, nationalities, or manner of expression.

Take, for instance, the aspect of Karma Yoga concerning the performance of acts of selfless love towards all people, no matter who they may be. This principle of selfless love can be illustrated by the words of Cicero: '*Beneficus est quinon sua sed alterius causa benigne facit*—He is beneficent who acts kindly not for his own sake, but for another's.' The Yogic concept that the goal of all mankind is Knowledge is embodied in the words of Socrates: 'There is one good thing only, knowledge, and one evil thing, ignorance.' The great German poet, Goethe, understood the futility of seeking praise or the fruits of one's actions. '*Die Tat ist alles; nichts der Ruhm*—The deed is everything, fame is nothing.'

One could find endless quotations but the above three will demonstrate my point that Yoga is not an esoteric cult but a perfectly feasible way of life, of thought, of action which takes in Universal Truth by means of a singularly high standard of conduct.

Let us consider, now, the power of the spoken and written word. Few people think of the power of words when they speak, and few who are not writers or lawyers think carefully before they commit anything to paper. To use words well is part of Karma Yoga, for words are actions, and actions inevitably have reactions. So the student of Karma Yoga has to take great care that no base or unkind words pass his lips, even if he has been harmed by another person. The harmful action itself carries its own Karma with it and therefore needs no help from anyone else! The student of Karma Yoga must also be careful with the words of others. Kindness and reasonableness will open your ears to what others really *mean*, not merely what they say. The two can be very different, as many people know to their cost. The study of Karma Yoga helps one to distinguish sincerity from insincerity, truth from falsehood, and this can be of great help in inter-personal relationships in everyday life. Karma Yoga makes great demands on its followers but it is nothing if not practical.

Those of my pupils who have studied Karma Yoga with me have, on the whole, found some difficulty in understanding the close connection between good and evil, and have been daunted by the notion that no action can be wholly pure, nor wholly impure. In every action there is the inevitable association of good and evil. It is part of Life itself. But let me bring this from the general to the particular. Let us suppose that a man commits a theft. If he is found out and imprisoned for his crime, one could still find some good in his action if the theft brought him to the eventual realization of his own base action and so to the determination not to repeat it. One could apply this principle to all actions of a base nature, and conversely to all noble actions as well. For instance, a man might be a great scientist and discover the cure for some dread disease, bringing relief and benefit to thousands of suffering human beings. But if he has killed one small animal in his research, one single microbe even, there is this element of evil in all his good work. This is how things are and we cannot change them, and students of Karma Yoga must learn to accept this difficult association between good and evil as a fact of life.

Think, for instance, of fire: when we are cold there is no greater comfort than a warm fire or some form of heat. But if fire burns to warm us and to warm our food, it can also burn our cities, our forests, our ships. It gives life but it can also take life. So fire is neither wholly good nor wholly evil, but both. So is every element of nature. Without water no human being can live. But too much water ruins crops and causes starvation. Electricity when harnessed is a force for good but think of its terrible aspect in nature. And now in our twentieth century we have nuclear energy. Here is a power that can wipe out whole cities and destroy or maim thousands of human beings. But it can also drive great machines, with enormous benefit to mankind. If we view everything in this twofold way we begin to understand that good and evil can never be independent of each other.

Karma Yoga recognizes the nature of work, that it is a part of the foundation of nature and is never-ceasing, and the way of Karma Yoga is to plunge into the world of work and discover the secret of working without the desire for personal gain. That is the secret of work to be learned from the study of Karma Yoga. The goal of all the Yogas is freedom and in Karma Yoga that goal can be reached through selfless work. 'To work you have the right but not to the fruits thereof.'

In the Bhagavad Gita Krishna speaks on this subject to Arjuna:

Work with desire is verily far inferior to that performed with the mind undisturbed by thoughts of results. Therefore seek refuge in this evenness of mind. Wretched are they who act for results.

Endued with this evenness of mind one frees oneself in this life, alike from vice and virtue. Devote thyself, therefore, to this Karma Yoga. It is the very dexterity of work.

The meaning of the 'dexterity of work' is as follows: it is the nature of work to produce bondage. Karma Yoga is the dexterity of work because it not only robs work of its power to bind, but also transforms it into an efficient means towards freedom.

Krishna speaks further to Arjuna about Karma Yoga:

He who restraining the organs of action, sits revolving in the mind thoughts regarding objects of senses, he, of deluded understanding, is called a hypocrite.

But he who, controlling the senses by the mind, directs his organs of action to the path of work, he, O Arjuna, excels.

Do thou perform obligatory action; for action is superior to inaction; and even the bare maintenance of thy body would not be possible if thou art inactive.

The world is bound by actions other than those performed with a good motive; do thou, therefore, O Arjuna, perform action for good motives alone, devoid of desire for results.

To sum up this profound and fascinating, albeit difficult philosophy of Karma Yoga—it is the means by which the student learns how best to use action, all action, all thoughts, words, deeds, whether his own or those of others. Karma Yoga is the philosophy of work, of action, by which we may achieve that non-attachment to things, that abnegation of Self which is the highest plane of Yogic culture, and through which we can achieve peace. Every person we meet in our day-to-day lives offers us an opportunity to practise Karma Yoga and this is why, when it becomes more widely known in the Western world, it will doubtless be more acceptable to a wider section of the public than those Yogas which require one to work alone and in secret. People are the raw material of the would-be Karma Yogi. He cannot do without them, because Karma Yoga is a system of ethics designed towards the attainment of freedom through the incessant practice of unselfish action.

Non-attachment, renunciation of action, is hard to attain without performance of action; the wise man, the Karma Yogi, purified by devotion to action, finally attains peace.

The Bhagavad Gita

Chapter 11

COMMON SENSE ABOUT MEDITATION

Go far into the void, and there rest in quietness.
All things arise, and bloom in their time, and then they return to
their root.
Their returning is peace.

The Tao Te Ching XVI
Version by Juan Mascaró

THIS IS a controversial subject to say the least, and a sitting target for an unbelievable number of fallacies and misapprehensions which have long needed to be remedied.

Of the large number of people in the Western part of the world who want and need Yoga, I am continually surprised at how many there are who say they prefer to confine themselves to the practice of meditation and who ask endless questions about it; but by and large the main question is how they are to set about it.

So for these people, and all the others who want to know, here is a chapter which might have been called 'Meditation for Beginners', were it not for the amount of nonsense which has been, and still is, believed about it, and with which I shall deal as I go along.

First of all, what exactly *is* meditation? The short answer is that it is the endeavour to bring into the mind in its everyday state of activity (what in Yoga is called the waking consciousness), that which may be called the super-consciousness. In other words, meditation is the lower or bodily self reaching upwards to the ideal or higher Self.

Already we have reached the first stumbling-blocks. To some people the only tangible reality is the physical body and the material things which surround it, and what is called the soul or higher Self is a mere intellectual theory. And so, in my opinion, the first things which need to be learnt are the obstacles in the way of the would-be meditator. These are many but one can cut them down to a basic six, namely disease, pain, mental laziness, doubt, lethargy, and negative emotion.

I will deal with these in turn. Firstly we can take disease and pain together. An unhealthy person, or one in any kind of physical discomfort from a headache to indigestion, cannot successfully practise meditation—unless he happens to be a Ramakrishna that is, but how many people are! So first things first. A person who is ill or suffers from pain for any reason at all must first go to a teacher of Yoga to learn the disciplines of Hatha Yoga so that his body may regain its health; he will learn to gain control over it and the problem of the physical pain will thus disappear. I know there are people, indeed whole societies, who make sincere attempts to disregard the body altogether and who feel that 'one ought to be able to control the mind whatever the circumstances'.

Theoretically I suppose this is true, but in all the years I have been writing books and articles on Yoga I have always attempted to make it accessible to the ordinary Western man-in-the-street, the person who has to be at his or her desk at nine o'clock in the morning after travelling to work in an overcrowded train or bus; to the person who does a repetitive and soul-destroying job and who feels there is somehow 'something better' somewhere. I do not write about Yoga for saints, and people who can go away and live in the Himalayas, leaving all the cares and responsibilities of everyday living behind them.

So I am wholly convinced that disease and pain should be dealt with before meditation is attempted. It is by far the easiest course to take. Why do things the hard way? Disease and pain drag the body and the mind downwards, and what one is attempting to do in meditation is to draw the mind upwards.

What about mental laziness? This obstacle can only be overcome from within. No Yoga teacher can help those who are too lazy to practise, to persevere, to accept each failure as a challenge over which to triumph. Perfection in any kind of Yoga is never achieved without perseverence, and how one's character does show when it comes to mental laziness!

Doubt. Now this is a serious obstacle, and hard to overcome. Many students of Yoga go through a period of doubt to such an extent that it causes a complete mental block and they feel they have to give up meditation altogether. To people who have had this problem, and most do go through this phase to a greater or lesser degree, I can only say that it is a phase that will pass, if the student is prepared to persevere through it. Strangely enough, if the student is prepared to do this it seldom impedes progress for very long. Doubts arise in the minds of all thinking people, however strong their convictions, and a teacher can do a great deal here to strengthen the student's resolve.

Lethargy. This of course could be due to some sickness of the body, and Hatha Yoga is indicated here if this is the case. If, however, a state of apathy exists in a perfectly healthy body, then the student is not yet ready for the strenuous intellectual control required for successful meditation. Enthusiasm is one of the vital qualities necessary for meditation. Half-hearted stabs at it are more than futile.

Negative emotion. This is the greatest enemy of all students of Yoga. The mind churns over past conversations; one thinks of all the clever and witty things one might have said and did not; one remembers past hurts to one's pride and ego which arouse indignation and a desire to hit back. One worries about future events: will we make an impression, will we get that job, pass that examination, win that competition, and so on. The mind dwells fruitlessly on the might-have-been or on vague fears and anxieties, and so the mind becomes clouded with negative emotions such as anger, hate, fear, panic, even hysteria. Reality can fade before a tangle of negative emotion unless one tries to exercise some control over one's thoughts. If you give in to your negative emotion you will take a step backwards. If you replace it with some positive thought or action and accept what *is*, you have taken your first step in meditation.

Swami Vivekananda used to say that a man's mind is like a lake, the bed of which is the true Self; and that it is possible to see the bed of the lake only when the water is calm. If the water is muddy or impure in any way, or if it becomes agitated, the lake-bed is hidden. To discover the true Self, therefore, the state of Sattva (serenity) must be cultivated until the mind-lake becomes tranquil and clear. It is, the Swami said, the greatest manifestation of strength to be calm at will, to be in control of one's body and mind.

One of the greatest and most effective antidotes to fruitless indulgence in negative emotion is the relaxation of the body combined with slow deep breathing. As the muscles relax and tension leaves the body, it also begins to leave the mind, which gradually becomes calm and once more under one's control.

Having thus been made aware of the negative pull-backs which would-be students of meditation have to contend with, the student himself is more in a position to decide whether or not he can approach the first step in meditation with any degree of confidence.

The very first thing is to find what I have called a 'peace symbol'. This can take any form within the limits I shall indicate. It must be a tangible object and not merely an idea. A colour is not suitable, being too abstract. Nor will a piece of music be effective as music is essentially dynamic and the whole point about a 'peace symbol' is that it must not only be relatively immobile, but must also have an air of tranquillity about it. In shape it must be fairly simple and graceful, the more beautiful the better, and under no circumstances must it be connected in the student's mind with any disturbing or unpleasant incident. It must be, as is implicit in its name, a symbol of peace.

For the beginner who cannot think of a suitable 'peace symbol' within these limitations, I can make a few suggestions. A candle-flame is an ideal subject, being simple in outline and gentle in movement. It conveys a feeling of tranquillity yet has a brightness which is slightly hypnotic. Also the upward movement conveys exactly what is needed in meditation, which is to make the mind lift.

Other students may prefer a leaf from a favourite plant or tree, a flower, a simple geometrical shape, or the soft outlines of a sleeping animal.

Having decided on your 'peace symbol' you should keep it permanently, for gradually it will become for you not only the symbol of peace within your mind but an effective means of stilling agitated mind-states when calmness is of the utmost importance to you in your day-to-day dealings with other people and circumstances. In your home, in the office, driving your car, waiting in a traffic jam, writing an examination paper, dealing with an unruly classful of children —whatever your occupation may be, or whatever you happen to be doing at the time which may be causing annoyance and frustration, your 'peace symbol' will be with you whenever it is most needed.

So to sum up, find a suitable 'peace symbol', stick to it, and above all *remember to use it*. You would be surprised how many people go to the trouble of finding a really good symbol and then forget all about it as soon as things begin to go against them. So the next step is to cultivate the thought of your peace symbol until it becomes habitual. Try to make it the last thing you think about before you go to sleep at night, and the first as you awaken in the morning. During the waking hours try to remember that you have, and always have had, the ability to fix your mind on any subject you please, and as you remember this, fix your mind on your peace symbol.

If you are a 'naturally' restless or nervous person, you have probably been pursuing a damaging thought-habit for years. For some reason, most people find it easier to panic than to calm down and think reasonably. If you are one of these people then do not be impatient for any immediate results from your first attempts at meditation. Do not be surprised if you forget your carefully chosen peace symbol for days on end. It happens to most people.

Meditation is often divided into three stages; concentration, meditation, and contemplation. The first of these is by far the most difficult. It takes long and gradual practice. It takes patience. Above all it requires enormous mental effort.

So you have chosen your peace symbol, and now you have to learn to concentrate on it. It helps if you repeat, either aloud or inside your head, the ideas about it that pass through your mind. As an example let us take my white rose as the symbol. You say to yourself, 'This rose is white, but not chalky white. It looks almost green (or cream) in the centre. It reflects the light where the petals fold back. It is a large rose, and the darkness of its leaves emphasise its colour. The stalk is almost brown. The shape of the rose reminds me of a dancer's tutu. It has two drops of water on its petals . . .' and so on.

In this manner, the student learns by degrees to concentrate on his particular symbol, shutting out from his thoughts anything extraneous. With time and patience he will achieve some measure of concentration; the ideal, of course, is to be able, at will, to bring the peace symbol into the mind, hold it there for several seconds, and think of nothing else at all.

You might find it easier to reach this stage if you choose as a peace symbol something you can actually sit and look at until every detail is fixed in your mind. Then close your eyes, sit quietly, and bring your symbol into your mind's eye and 'fix' it in the space between your eyebrows. It will appear smaller than in its actual physical form, but will be an exact replica in all other respects.

Direct your thoughts onto your symbol and when they begin to stray away, lead them very carefully back again. This method requires constant practice, as does the other, but when you are accomplished at either method this first step in mental control will enter your everyday life as an effective means of dispelling anxiety, worry, and all those negative emotions that impede the mind's upward lift, that tranquillity of mind and calm control which is the aim of all

Yoga.

Having come as far as this a student could safely consider himself to have the qualities of perseverence necessary to the practice of meditation, and at this stage we can consider meditation itself. The following meditation will help to expand the student's consciousness. Let him consider all the beauties of nature that come to his mind; birds in flight; the rich brown of horses and cows; the lovely patterns and textures of wood; trees, flowers; the flood of pleasure at waking one morning to find a tree has blossomed overnight; sunlight on snow —is there any end to the beauties of nature? Let the student sit quite still and meditate on these things whenever he has a quiet moment. At this stage the mental control will seem considerably easier than the singleness of mind required in connection with the peace symbol.

After meditating upon the beauties of nature, the next stage is to meditate on all the masterpieces of art that have come from the hand of Man. Let the student meditate on great pictures and sculpture, on music and literature and poetry. Let him meditate on all the greatness of which the human mind is capable. With practice these meditations should never leave him, even in times of stress, because meditations helps to still the turmoil of our emotions, the restless activity of the brain, even under the most trying circumstances.

When the student can 'lift' his mind at will he can then be said to have reached the stage of contemplation. He will have grown more responsive to higher influences, and by contrast the lower things of which man is capable will become wholly distasteful. In such a way does meditation help to build character and help the individual to realize his latent potential.

Also, with the change in character and personality comes a change in outlook which in its turn helps to make life in general more pleasant and easy. As the inner life changes and becomes richer, so one creates around oneself an environment which reflects the inner peace. Inter-personal relationships consequently benefit, and so ultimately, the practice of meditation is not, as so many think, a selfish pursuit; on the contrary it is of benefit to others. And after all, is this not the aim of Yoga?

Chapter 12

A COMPARISON BETWEEN GREEK AND INDIAN PHILOSOPHY

Every soul of man has in the way of nature looked on True Being;
this was the condition of her passing into the form of man. But all
souls do not easily recall the things of the other world; they may
have seen them for a short time only, or they may have been unfor-
tunate in their earthly lot, and, having had their hearts turned to
unrighteousness through some corrupting influence, they may have
lost the memory of the holy things which once they saw. Few only
retain an adequate remembrance of them; and they, when they
see here any image of that other world, are rapt in amazement.

PLATO *Phaedrus*
Translated by Jowett

IT WAS once pointed out by an English orientalist, and quite rightly
I believe, how impossible it is to study the Vedanta or the Bhagavad
Gita without coming to the conclusion that the ancient Greeks, of
which Socrates, Plato, Aristotle and Pythagoras are the most
eminent, derived their theories quite independently from the same
source as did the Vedic sages of ancient India, even though the
latter ante-date the Greek school by many centuries.

This leads anyone with an enquiring mind to delve deeper in order
to be able to compare the one school of thought with the other. The
ancient Greeks upheld the theory of One Absolute Existence as
opposed to that of the many; or, as the Ionian philosopher, Anaxa-
goras (possibly the teacher of Socrates) puts it, 'a Supreme
Intelligence, the most pure and subtle of all things.' If we look into
the Mundaka Upanishad we read about 'Absolute Existence and
Absolute Knowledge.'

Both schools of thought give a clear picture of an ultimate goal of
unity towards which all philosophies (and of course religions)
inevitably tend. The word Yoga itself means unity, conjunction,
oneness, the implication being with an Absolute Existence.

Because of the vastness and the engrossing nature of the present subject one would prefer to write a whole book on it instead of one chapter. But space is seldom on the side of the writer, even the writer of books, and so I will have to be content with confining myself to a comparison between the theories of one of the Greek philosophers and those of the ancient Indian sages. This, even so, leaves me ample scope to develop my thesis that human ideals belong, and always have belonged, to every school of thought and therefore to every individual. And in finding just one Greek philosopher my choice inevitably falls on Plato. Why? Subjectively (my writer's prerogative!) because I love to read him; I like his dynamic writing style, and to follow the impeccable logic of that great mind seems to me as rare a delight as listening to the last five quartets of Beethoven. It is a wholly satisfying experience and if one can understand and enjoy the fruits of human minds of the order of Plato's and Beethoven's one is, I believe, privileged. Objectively I choose Plato because of the dialogue form of his writings, because many of India's greatest books, including the Upanishads, the Bhagavad Gita and the Last Message of Sri Krishna are also written in this form. This similarity makes comparison that much easier for those of my readers whose interest and imagination may be caught by the examples I shall represent here and who may wish to find more for themselves.

So I have chosen Plato and I quote here from *The Republic*.

This is my counsel; let us believe that the soul is immortal, and able to bear all ill and all good, and let us always keep to the upward way.

Compare this with the words of Lord Krishna in the Bhagavad Gita:

I shall describe that which has to be known, knowing which one attains to immortality. It is called neither being nor non-being . . . The Light even of lights, It is said to be beyond darkness; Knowledge, and the One Thing to be known, the Goal of knowledge, dwelling in the hearts of all.

And again:

The Imperishable is the Supreme Brahman. Its dwelling in each individual body is called Adhyatma; the offering in virtuous works which causes the genesis and support of beings is called Karma.

This last word perhaps requires clarification. According to the Bhagavad Gita the working out of one's Karma, according to the law of one's own being, is the way to the highest knowledge. In other words Plato's 'Upward way'.

We can further compare Lord Krishna's words with those from Plato's *Republic*:

> That calm man who is the same in pain and pleasure, whom these cannot disturb, alone is capable to attain to immortality.

The implication here is that worldly things are in their nature impermanent and only the Self is changeless and indestructible.

This word Self appears constantly in both Greek and Indian philosophy and it is also interesting to note the great psychologist Carl Jung's use of this word. His concept of the Self, superior to the ego, represents in his view the individual in his totality. And note his choice of the word in the title of his book, *The Undiscovered Self*; and that in his work, *The Development of Personality*, he writes, 'There is no personality without definiteness, wholeness and ripeness.' All this sounds like Yoga, which is exactly what it is. Carl Jung is known to have been interested in both Indian and Buddhist philosophy.

And as the great Jung paid Yoga the compliment of adopting one of its most vital terms, so there can never have been a true Yoga teacher or a philosopher who did not have a thoroughgoing knowledge of depth psychology or, before that term came into being, of the human mind in its complexity and totality.

And the word psychology comes from the Greek *psukhē* meaning soul, mind, breath or life. Which brings me back to Plato. He was uncompromising in his belief in the correlation between the highest type of conduct and the highest type of knowledge. And this knowledge he said can be gained only in that region that lies beyond mere physical perception or intellectualizing. In the last book of the *Republic* he writes:

> Our recent argument and the other proofs compel us to the conclusion that the soul is immortal. But if we are to see it as it is in truth, we ought not to see it as we do at present, polluted by the

association of the body . . .

And further on he writes:

We must turn our eyes, Glaucon, to the soul's love of wisdom, and after what company she strives led on by her kinship to the divine and immortal and that which ever is.

These examples echo the injunction of the Vedas that

Truth cannot be attained either by mere study, by intellectual reasoning or by constantly listening to it. That the man who has not rejected evil conduct, whose senses lack control, and whose mind is not at ease, can never attain Truth.

In the Bhagavad Gita we find a parallel thought as applied to the individual. Lord Krishna says:

He whose heart is steadfastly engaged in the practice of Yoga, who looks everywhere with the eyes of equality, seeing the Self in all beings and all beings in the Self . . . that one is highly esteemed.

Both the Indian philosophers and Plato lay great emphasis on the distinction between the spiritual and the physical.

'The soul is the divine and the body mortal,' writes Plato.

'These bodies are perishable but the dwellers in these bodies are eternal, indestructible and impenetrable,' says Lord Krishna in the Gita.

'If we would have pure knowledge of anything, we must be quit of the body, and the soul in herself must behold all things in themselves.' This is Socrates speaking in Plato's dialogue, *Phaedo*.

The Brihadaranyaka Upanishad, one of the eleven great books which form the closing portion of Vedic literature, expounds with much rational argument the Unity of Being and the inherent divinity and purity of the human soul. In Book Five of the *Republic* Plato discriminates with great clarity between *opinion* and *real knowledge*.

Knowledge is correlative to the existent and ignorance therefore to the non-existent. Opinion is something more obscure than knowledge, but more luminous than ignorance.

This is illustrated by the famous allegory of the cave in Book Seven of the *Republic*, in which Plato shows us how easy it is for Man, living the life of a prisoner in a cave and able to see only the shadows of things, to regard these as the only realities. And that naturally he would be puzzled if told that what he sees are mere phantoms. And if taken from his cave (of ignorance) into the light of the sun, would he not at first be so dazzled as to be unable to see clearly the reality around him?

And so here the two philosophies meet, the Indian and the Greek, in their concept of a Self or soul which is indestructible, and of a state of Pure Knowledge which this Self can attain. Both the Indian and the Greek philosophers concerned themselves with those subjects about which man has always been most curious and most vehement. And one has the unmistakable conviction that all these men had truths to tell and a vision that is as difficult to establish in words as it is rare and, to most ordinary men, barely comprehensible.

Yet we believe Plato because he was able to write about his vision with such passion and authority, and we believe the Indian sages when they tell us, so often and so consistently, in all their great books, that Man is in bondage so long as he remains in ignorance of his true Self. Because dimly we too have sometimes understood, seen a vision for perhaps only a second, and then lost it again. But these brief glimpses we never forget.

Another aspect of the correlation between Greek and Indian thought is the attitude of both to ignorance and knowledge. Let us give Socrates, Plato's great teacher, the floor for a moment. 'You must bear with me, dear Phaedrus—I am so fond of learning,' he says with prodigious understatement in the dialogue *Phaedrus*; and in *The Apology* he says:

Are you not ashamed of caring so much for the making of money and for reputation and for honour? Will you not think or care about wisdom and truth, and the perfection of your souls?

And now let us hear the boy, Alcibiades in his speech in honour of Socrates in the dialogue, *The Symposium*.

I have heard Pericles and other great orators, and thought they spoke well, but I never had any similar feeling [as when Socrates spoke]; my soul was not stirred by them, nor was I angry at the thought of my own slavish state.

Socrates, as we know him through the dialogues of Plato, had a passion for knowledge, and while insisting on his own ignorance he never ceased his striving to convince others of theirs. His quarrel was never with people but with error and through Plato we know of his extraordinary precision in his use of terms. In the dialogue, *Lysis* he says,

> In matters of which we have knowledge all people will trust us, whether Greeks or barbarians, men or women . . . With regard to matters, on the other hand, into which we have acquired no insight, no one will ever allow us to act as we think proper . . . and we ourselves in these matters shall be subject to others. If therefore you acquire knowledge, my dear Lysis, all men will be friendly to you, and all will be attached to you; for you will be useful and good.

The views of Socrates and Plato regarding knowledge and ignorance were upheld, centuries later, by another intellectual giant, Swami Vivekananda who echoed the Vedas and the Upanishads in his view that ignorance is the source of all the world's evil.

In the Rig Veda Man is conscious of a spiritual transgression; there has been a sin of ignorance, and Man sings to Varuna,

> May the stream of my life flow into the river of righteousness. Loose the bonds of sin that bind me. Let not the thread of my song be cut while I sing.

In the Isa Upanishad we are told:

> He who knows both knowledge and action, with action overcomes death and with knowledge reaches immortality.

In the Gita we read,

> Light, fire and darkness are the three constituents of nature. Darkness which is born of ignorance darkens the souls of all men.

In Chapter Three of the Gita Lord Krishna tells the warrior Prince,

Arjuna,

Wisdom is clouded by desire, the everpresent enemy of the wise.

And in Chapter Four:

Some, faithful to austere vows, offer their practice of Yoga, their
studies and their knowledge . . .
When wisdom is thine, Arjuna, never more shalt thou be in confusion . . . And even if thou wert the greatest of sinners, with the
help of the bark of wisdom thou shalt cross the sea of evil.

Again from the Gita:

Knowledge is enveloped in ignorance, hence do beings get
deluded.

Though my concern in this chapter is with a comparison between
Plato and Indian philosophy, those views of which I have given
examples were by no means confined to the great thinkers of Greece
and the Vedanta. To quote just a few illustrations from the rest of
the world's wisdom I naturally give first place to Confucius, and the
Gautama Buddha.

Shall I teach thee what is wisdom? To know what we know, and
know what we do not know.

CONFUCIUS

Remember what I have said, I have said; and what I have not said,
I have not said. And why have I not answered certain questions?
Because they are not profitable, they lead not to peace, and to
wisdom.

The Gautama Buddha

Two things fill the mind with ever new and increasing admira-
tion and awe, the more and the deeper we consider them: the
heavens above with their myriad stars, and the moral law within.

KANT *Critique of Practical Reason*

He who is strong and yet chooses gentleness is like unto a lake

138

that lies low, but which receives the waters of the high mountains.
The Tao Te Ching XXVIII

We are convinced that our Torah agrees with Greek philosophy, which substantiates with convincing proofs the contention that man's conduct is entirely in his own hands, that no compulsion is exerted, and that no *external* influence is brought to bear on him that constrains him to be either virtuous or vicious . . .

MAIMONIDES

If men believed that the mind perishes with the body, they would return to their own inclinations . . . Such a course appears to me not less absurd than if a man, because he does not believe that he can by wholesome food sustain his body forever, should wish to cram himself with poisons; or if because he believes that the mind is not eternal and immortal, he should prefer to be out of mind altogether, and to live without the use of reason.

SPINOZA *Ethics*

To endure all things with an equable and peaceful mind not only brings with it many blessings to the soul; but it also enables us, in the midst of our difficulties, to have a clear judgement about them, and to minister the fitting remedy for them.

ST JOHN OF THE CROSS
The Ascent of Mount Carmel

> Anger hast thou not forgotten,
> Nor falsehood;
> Then why hast thou forgotten Truth.

GURU NANAK *(Sikhism)*

> Why so large cost, having so short a lease,
> Dost thou upon thy fading mansion spend?
> Shall worms, inheritors of this excess,
> Eat up thy charge?

SHAKESPEARE

The Shakespeare brings me to a further point. Neither Plato nor the Vedic sages condemned the body or regarded it as evil in itself. It only becomes so when we cease to regard it as anything more than a mere instrument. In different language both schools of thought express the same viewpoint.

This body is mortal and always held by death. It is the abode of that Self which is immortal and without body. When in the body, by thinking this body is I, and I am this body, the Self is held by pleasure and pain. When free of the body then neither pleasure nor pain touches it.

CHANDOGYA UPANISHAD

And Socrates, in Plato's *Phaedo*, speaks thus to his friends:

Do you think that the lover of knowledge ought to care about the pleasures of eating and drinking? And will he think much of the other ways of indulging the body? Would you not say that he is entirely concerned with the soul and not with the body? He would like, as far as he can, to be quit of the body and turn to the soul.

It is interesting that both ancient India and ancient Greece, though their systems of physical culture evolved in very different ways, had a physical ideal which was a man of perfect equilibrium in body and mind. In Greece the physical ideal was a gymnast or athlete, in India he was an adept at Hatha Yoga. But both Vedic literature and Plato's writings warn us of the futility of making a goal out of that which is a mere instrument. To do so inhibits the original function which the instrument might have served.

It is fortunate, however, that Man has a tendency to progress from the world of matter to that of mind and this process is enhanced as each individual grows older.

Know the Supreme Self as the Lord of the chariot, and the body as the chariot. Know also the intellect to be the charioteer, mind the reins, and the senses are called the horses.

KATHA UPANISHAD
Translated by Juan Mascaró

The senses are said to be superior to the body; the mind is superior to the senses; the intellect is superior to the mind; and that which is superior to the intellect is the Self.

Bhagavad Gita Chapter 3

140

The wise one, even though in the body, is not of it, like a man awakened from dream.

The Last Message of Sri Krishna

There are those who insist that there is no point in reading and studying anything so ancient as Vedic literature or the dialogues of Plato and the works of the other great Greek philosophers, but in my opinion there are few bodies of work which repay study better and which are more relevant to the 1970s. Our present age is one of violent change in which the foundations of old beliefs are breaking down. So it was in the time of Plato, and so to read him is to re-examine our contemporary problems in perspective. Everything in the 1970s is under scrutiny: human relationships, religion and the nature of belief, philosophy and politics, to name but a few fundamental issues vital to every individual. But there is no topic of importance which is now under scrutiny to which Plato did not apply his mind. And Vedic literature is a blend of idealism, philosophical enquiry, practical wisdom and common sense which outlines a way of life which could well be the answer to many of the problems which beset the world today. Vedic literature is, as Plato is, timeless.

But still, you may object, Plato was only a Utopian and so were the Vedic sages. And that is true enough. But what was the Buddha, what was Christ, what were St John and Spinoza and William Blake? Have not all great thinkers been Utopians and as such were they not revolutionaries? Were those ancient visionaries and prophets not practical men after all? It gives one cause to think, doesn't it? Which is why the ancient Greek philosophers and the Vedic sages can still speak to us across the centuries. Wisdom and Truth, after all, take no account of time.

Chapter 13

SWAMI VIVEKANANDA, YOGA'S MODERN INTELLECTUAL GIANT

And I have felt
A presence that disturbs me with the joy
Of elevated thoughts; a sense sublime
Of something far more deeply interfused,
Whose dwelling is the light of setting suns,
And the round ocean and the living air,
And the blue sky, and in the mind of man:
A motion and a spirit, that impels
All thinking things, all objects of all thought,
And rolls through all things . . .

WILLIAM WORDSWORTH

WHEN travelling in America the Swami, being dark-skinned, was taken for a Negro in certain towns in the Deep South, and was consequently refused admission to 'white' hotels. He did not mention to anyone that he was not of African blood but simply and gratefully availed himself of the society and hospitality that was offered—that of the coloured people. Later, when the local magnates learned how the Swami had been treated, they rushed to apologize for what they considered a grave insult to him. 'But why,' they asked, 'why did you say nothing?' 'What, rise at the expense of another!' the Swami answered: 'I did not come to earth for that.'

To the many who love the Swami already this anecdote will come as no surprise. To the many who have yet to learn about him, it speaks volumes about the man.

He was born Narendraneth Dutta on January 12th, 1863 and lived until 1902—just over thirty-nine years, and yet, because of those few years, India was never to be the same again. He was without doubt an intellectual giant, but he was much more than that. He was a great teacher and orator, and his teachings span a wide field from logic, philosophy and reason to science, ethics and religion.

Basically what he wanted, and what the aim of his whole life was dedicated to, was a synthesis of all that is best in Indian and Western thought so that both cultures should benefit. He wanted India to learn from the West the capacity for hard work, organization, and scientific achievement. And he felt that the West had much to gain from the religion and spirituality of the people of India, and that what was badly needed was the Indian's innate sense of peace and serenity. In the West life was characterized by mad activity, materialism, ambition, frustration, and a general lack of equilibrium. If this was so when the Swami lived, how much more is it true now in the 1970s, and we can benefit that much more from the Swami's words, if only we would stop to read them, and to act upon them.

It is far from easy to evaluate how far Swami Vivekananda influenced the synthesis of the Indian and the Western intellectual outlook in view of the fact of Mahatma Gandhi's enormous political influence and achievements. One could say, I believe, that Gandhi, less liberal minded, was less inclined to give recognition to a synthesis of Indian and Western thought, and because of this one cannot help wondering if, in the fullness of time, his work will be overshadowed by that of Swami Vivekananda, who at the moment is the less famous man outside India.

Basically Gandhi was all for India, while Swami Vivekananda's teachings were essentially universal. The Swami took the philosophy of the Vedanta, one of the greatest intellectual systems known to mankind, and re-interpreted it in terms understandable both to India and the Western world.

His ideas on education, for instance, were, to say the least, thought-provoking. He believed that all knowledge is within the brain of man and requires only awakening, and that this awakening, and *not* instruction, is the real function of the teacher.

Compare this viewpoint with Plato's dialogue, *Meno*, in which Socrates examines the origin of knowledge. 'Every soul,' he says, 'has a seed which may germinate into all knowledge.' And to illustrate his point he elicits rudimentary geometry from a completely illiterate slave, meanwhile saying to his friend, Meno,

I shall only *ask* him, and not teach him, and he shall share the inquiry with me; and you shall watch and see if you can find me telling or explaining anything to the boy, instead of eliciting his opinion.

143

And further on in the dialogue Socrates says,

> If there have always been true thoughts in him which need only
> be *awakened* into knowledge by putting questions to him, his soul
> must have always possessed this knowledge . . .

The concept of this *a priori* knowledge is by no means confined
to Plato and Vivekananda, indeed it has always been accepted by
many of the world's greatest philosophers. One wonders, therefore,
why it is not used as a basis for the education of children in the
1970s instead of the more conventional methods of teaching. If it
were, the results might well be revolutionary.

The Swami felt that teachers are too much carried away by words
and that in a torrent of words the essence of what is being taught is
lost. But for all his knowledge, his original thinking, and his uniquely 'modern' ideas, we must not lose sight of the fact that the
Swami was a monk, a religious man, and that this religion permeates
all that he has to say to us.

He lived his life according to the pantheistic principles set down
in the Bhagavad Gita and believed implicitly in its doctrine of service
to one's fellow men. 'Because if a spark of divinity dwells in all men,
then he who serves all men serves God' was the way he reasoned.
And of course the same idea of service to one's fellow men is all over
Christianity, Judaism, Hinduism, Islam, Sikhism, indeed all the
great religions of the world.

> Be with us, as You were with our fathers, and give us strength
> and courage, that we may live and work in Your name to establish
> peace, and justice, love and fellowship among all men.
>
> *Judaism*

> Benevolence works and asks nothing.
>
> *Taoism*

> One man, when he has done a service to another, is ready to set
> it down to his account as a favour conferred.
> Another is not ready to do this, but still, in his own mind, he
> thinks of the man as his debtor, and he knows what he has done.
> A third, in a manner, does not even know what he has done, but
> he is like a vine which has produced grapes, and seeks for nothing

more after it has produced its proper fruit. So a man when he has done a good act, does not call out for others to come and see, but he goes on to another act as a vine goes on to produce again the grapes in season.

Marcus Aurelius

It is the most difficult thing in the world, to work and not care for the result, to help a man and never think that he ought to be grateful, to do some good work and at the same time never look to see whether it brings you name or fame, or nothing at all . . .

A man must remember that his life is for the service of God and the poor.

SWAMI VIVEKANANDA

The Swami, after wandering, mostly on foot, through the length and breadth of India, and performing intense spiritual disciplines, reached Kanyakumari in 1892 where at last he discovered the real purpose of his existence, namely the regeneration of India, its religion, its culture, its intellectual standards. And he was determined that this 'awakening as if from a long sleep' of India was to be of benefit to the whole of mankind, and not confined to the people of his own country.

And so, like the Buddha, two thousand five hundred years before him, the Swami emerged from his meditations and, filled with resolve, arrived in Madras where the period of his obscurity ended forever. In September, 1893, he attended the Parliament of Religions in Chicago, where his speeches were characterized by a tremendous force of conviction, by his intense humanity and sincerity, and by his broad and entirely modern outlook. His message was simple, namely the inherent divinity in Man and his capacity for infinite intellectual evolution.

His speeches were brilliant—he was a great orator—and his closing one proclaimed that every religion in the world has produced men and women of exalted character and that 'harmony and not dissension' should and one day would be the keynote of every world faith.

His words were to be, in a sense, prophetic. The Chicago Parliament of Religions is remembered because of the dynamic character of Vivekananda, and it in turn introduced him to the American public. Both in the United States, and when he returned to India in

1897, he emphasized the greatness of the Vedanta philosophy and mankind's need for making spirituality, as opposed to materialism, the basis of every national programme.

Apart from his brilliant lectures and teachings wherever he went, the Swami made another gift to India and the rest of the world in the founding of a monastic Order bearing the name of his teacher, Sri Ramakrishna, who had died in 1886.

In 1899, Swami Vivekananda established the Ramakrishna Math at Belur in Bengal and in 1909 it was registered under the Societies' Registration Act of 1860 as the Ramakrishna Mission.

Throughout all his activity in connection with the establishment of the Mission, the Swami's one overriding idea was to make the Vedanta *practical*, how to bridge the gulf between spirituality and modern everyday living. Life demands, as the Swami well knew, a feasible reconciliation of these two opposing factors; and this is where his intellectual genius was brought fully into play. His formulation of practical, living Vedanta lies in his famous doctrine of service, that is, by all work becoming selfless, life itself can become a form of worship, therefore to work in the right frame of mind can become a form of prayer.

The aims and objects of the Ramakrishna Mission are embodied in the following extracts from the Memorandum of Association.

1. To impart and promote the study of Vedanta and its principles as propounded by Sri Ramakrishna and practically illustrated by the example of his own life, and of comparative Theology in its widest application.

2. To impart and promote the study of the arts, sciences and industries.

The Ramakrishna Mission has now been in existence for over sixty years and from humble beginnings it has grown to be a worldwide organization whose Centres establish essential points of contact between people of different races and beliefs. The work of the Mission in the Western world is mainly the dissemination of the universal principles of the Vedanta and of true ideas about India and her ancient culture.

Swami Vivekananda had the insight to see all religions as Man's endeavour to reach out above and beyond the limitations of his physical existence and his material surroundings, towards a greater and more permanent Reality. Harmony of religions is as much a need of the 1970s as it was when the Swami lived. He believed that it was essential to the peace and progress of mankind; and that intolerance, bigotry, and sectarianism were the cause of all the strife in the world. Was he not only too right?

And despite the enormous changes in the scientific and intellectual climate since the Swami lived, some of the world problems to which he applied his great intellect, and his solutions to them, are highly relevant to the 1970s. There is much neurosis in the West, there are wars in every part of the globe, we seem to live with fear and a sense of frustration. Would it not be common sense to think again about what the Swami had to teach us?

We cannot all be Vivekanandas but we can at least see his life example as an ideal towards which we can all strive. Obviously we cannot find a hard-and-fast guide in his actions and words as to how to conduct our own lives. He was in his way unique. He was an original thinker. He was full of practical common sense as few men are or have ever been. And in his life there was no inherent conflict between faith and reason, between action and meditation, between science and religion, as in most other people's lives.

He never ceased in his search for a temporal existence regulated by ethical principles, and he *lived* the Bhagavad Gita to such an extent that this ancient book has found, in this modern day and age, a dynamic expression in the life of a man who is one of the finest in India's spiritual heritage.

Chapter 14

THE YOGIC ATTITUDE TOWARDS WOMEN

God is thy law, thou mine; to know no more
Is woman's happiest knowledge and her praise.
MILTON *Paradise Lost*

AT VARIOUS times in the history of human culture, women have rebelled against the imposition of what is in effect man-made slavery. Their rebellions have been, at various times, effective to a greater or lesser degree, but women had little chance of real emancipation so long as men were in charge of the world's goods. And even now, in the so-called 'enlightened' 1970s the majority of adults still take for granted the myth of women's intellectual inferiority and children are indoctrinated with this false assumption in the vital formative years of their lives.

Yet few men know that there are large areas of the world where women are regarded as the dominant sex, and still fewer are aware of the fact that only a few thousand years ago in the highly developed agricultural civilizations of ancient Greece and Egypt, the system was matriarchal and women ruled the world as men rule it today. In ancient Egypt the child derived its name from its mother rather than its father. Men even wore cosmetics while women were out running the world's business, abjuring both cosmetics as absurd and their husbands for their pettiness and gossip!

This would seem to disprove the idea of masculine and feminine character traits, as such, even though the roles have been so completely reversed within historical times. In actuality what we call 'masculine' signifies that which belongs to the dominant sex, and 'feminine' conversely means that which belongs to the subjugated one.

But do we have to be a Plato or an Aristotle to argue that if the inferiority of women were a natural and universal truth, there would be no laws needed, no social conventions needed, to keep women in their so-called 'place', or any age-old conspiracy (whether conscious

148

or not) to prevent them from regaining their former dominant position. Do we, after all, need laws to prevent an imbecile from becoming Prime Minister?

Competition between the masculine and feminine is essentially a human vice, the product of Man's highly developed brain. There is no such competition in the animal kingdom. Some psychiatrists would say that man/woman competition is the product of the man's fallacious interpretation of his natural place in the scheme of things, the result of a profound inferiority complex, which compels him to find a scapegoat for his own shortcomings. This is a fascinating point, and I am tempted to develop it further but space—even in a book—is never, as I have said, on the writer's side. So perhaps I will deal with it in my next book on Yoga.

In view of the brief outline I have given of the subjugation of women in historical times, is it surprising that so many neuroses of our present day and age can be traced directly to the attempt of intelligent women to establish their social equality and usefulness and, in many cases their superiority? The unnatural imposition of masculine dominance has resulted in two distinct types of female psychology: the 'slave mentality' and the 'rebel mentality'. Of the latter category one can see some women going too far in the opposite direction, becoming positively aggressive with their emancipation. Needless to say, a middle course is the one to aim for not only according to Yoga but to common sense.

The problem, though, with these male/female competitions is that they preclude satisfactory relationships between men and women and lead to appalling conflicts and unhappiness, neuroses, and marital tragedy. No intelligent woman who has had to live her life as a glorified charwoman because the (often unconscious) vanity of her husband would not allow her competition with him outside the home, will fail to understand the havoc caused by the patriarchal tradition in our present-day culture, or fail to deplore it because of its effect on mental health.

Leaving aside the minority of women who have been able to make their intelligence felt in the world (as this book goes to Press the Prime Minister of India is a woman and so is the Prime Minister of Israel), we may well ask ourselves why women in general have to do the world's menial work simply because they are female. And we may also wonder why more people cannot see that the belligerent drive for personal prestige on the part of men must inevitably disfigure their relationships with their female counterparts and result in unhappiness on both sides.

If we turn now to the culture of India and analyse why it has endured for thousands of years, although sometimes having had to survive long periods of darkness, we see that it is due to the rock-like stability of its foundations worked out by its early philosophers. One of the most significant of these foundations is the ideal of the innate divinity of mankind, this ideal being of immense value in Indian inter-personal relationships from which is derived India's social and cultural progress.

Naturally, among the man human relationships, that between a man and his wife is the most important. Indeed it is quite possible to judge the progress of any society or culture by the status accorded to women. It will no doubt surprise many that the present status of women in the 1970s is at a stage which had *already been passed* in the very earliest days of recorded Indian history. The Rig Veda represents woman as man's equal in both religious and civic matters. The Vedic woman is depicted as the companion and helpmeet of man.

In the Upanishads we find the idea of man and woman as equal halves of a divine unity, and the writing here is profoundly serious. But the very same idea is to be found in Plato's dialogue, *The Symposium*, in terms which are highly comic. I refer to the speech of Aristophanes who is, of course, the great clown of Greek literature. The setting of *The Symposium* is a banquet, after which a group of learned men are discussing the nature of love. I think the Aristophanes speech is worth quoting at some length because, although its terms are so different from those of the Upanishads, the ideas correspond so closely.

> First let me treat of the nature and state of man; for the original human nature was not like the present, but different. In the first place, the sexes were originally three in number, not two as they are now; there was man, woman, and the union of the two, having a name corresponding to this double nature; this once had a real existence, but is now lost, and the name only is preserved as a term of reproach. In the second place, the primeval man was round and had four hands and four feet, back and sides forming a circle, one head with two faces, looking opposite ways, set on a round neck and precisely alike: also four ears, and the remainder to

correspond. When he had a mind he could walk as men now do, and he could also roll over and over at a great rate, leaning on his four hands and four feet, eight in all, like tumblers going over and over with their legs in the air; this was when he wanted to run fast. Now there were these three sexes, because the sun, moon, and earth are three; and the man was originally the child of the sun, the woman of the earth, and the man-woman of the moon, which is made up of sun and earth, and they were all round and moved round and round like their parents. Terrible was their might and strength, and the thoughts of their hearts were great, and they made an attack upon the gods; doubt reigned in the councils of Zeus and of the gods. Should they kill them and annihilate the race with thunderbolts, as they had done the giants, then there would be an end of the sacrifice and worship which men offered to them; but, on the other hand, the gods could not suffer their insolence to be unrestrained. At last, after a good deal of reflection, Zeus discovered a way. He said, 'I have a notion which will humble their pride and mend their manners; they shall continue to exist, but I will cut them in two and then they will be diminished in strength and increased in numbers; this will have the advantage of making them more profitable to us. They shall walk upright on two legs, and if they continue insolent and won't be quiet, I will split them again and they shall hop about on a single leg.

He spoke and cut men in two; and as he cut them one after another, he bade Apollo give the face and the half of the neck a turn in order that the man might contemplate the section of himself: this would teach him a lesson of humility. He was also to heal their wounds and compose their forms . . .

After the division the two parts of man, each desiring his other half, came together, and threw their arms about one another eager to grow into one, and would have perished from hunger without ever making an effort, because they did not like to do anything apart; and when one of the halves died and the other survived, the survivor sought another mate and clung to that.

There is more of this comic material, but the above will serve to prove my point. To get away from humour, the spiritual view of man and woman which we find in the Upanishads is the very rock upon which the Indian cultural edifice stands. India has always upheld, in theory at least, the spiritual equality of man and woman. In practice, however, it has been a different story since the Vedic age. Even so, Indian *thought* has always equated woman's destiny with man's, that is the lifelong search for spiritual purity. Throughout Indian history we read of the right of women as well as men, to scale the heights of spirituality.

To return to modern psychology for a moment, we find that both it, and Indian historical thinkers consider the ideal man/woman relationship to be one of 'mature dependence', in other words an alliance where each partner is equally dependent upon the other while maintaining his and her own individuality.

The fact that in the last fifteen hundred years Indian women have lost more and more of their freedom and in consequence have become more and more dominated by their menfolk is largely due to the disturbed social conditions which lie within the province of the historian and the sociologist and which are too complex (added to the ever-present problem of space) for me to elaborate upon here. Fifteen hundred years is a long time, time enough for the personality of Indian women to be considerably diminished, as Swami Vivekananda often pointed out in his speeches.

Fortunately for Indian women, things have improved in India since the Swami's lifetime. Though there remains much room for improvement—a state which will last for many years to come—nevertheless India has striven to restore the social balance between men and women, with some success.

So how are we to view the Indian woman of the 1970s? In theory at least she is free to develop her intelligence to its highest potential and, what is perhaps more important, she is free to consider herself more a man's comrade than his inferior and to express her views and opinions freely. In the ideal marriage which is becoming more and more prevalent in modern India, both partners equally value each other's advice, loyalty and companionship. In no way is there any question of competition between man and wife and Indians in general feel that psychologically this is a more healthy state of affairs than that which prevails in the West.

But we cannot lose sight of the fact that this change for the better in India has been a very gradual one and has, in fact, taken several centuries to come about. Old habits and customs die hard, even in a spiritually orientated land like India. And of course there has been a corresponding change in the attitude of the Indian man of the

1970s. When he looks for a wife he tends now to want his equal in intelligence and social outlook. No longer does he look for a glorified housekeeper and child nurse with a pretty face. He looks for a woman who will be a true companion to him, with the strength of character to share his responsibilities and the vicissitudes of his life.

These changes have made marriage in India, in the present decade, a joint adventure with the accent on equality. Swami Vivekananda considered that a thriving and forward-looking society is built on a harmonious adjustment of duties and rights between husband and wife and not, as we find all too often in the West, competition between them. But perhaps the greatest lesson that India has to teach the West is the spiritual value accorded to women, an elevation which enables the Indian woman to lead a fuller, more satisfying life on every level.

According to Indian culture of the present day, the ideal of motherhood can be the highest goal of spirituality in woman. It is interesting that, to the Hindu, God is the mother of all creation and that Hindu children are brought up to regard all females as manifestations of the One Divine Mother. One's mind is drawn irresistibly to Erda, the Earth Mother, in Wagner's *Der Ring des Nibelungen*. The composer himself described Erda as 'the eternal woman possessed of all the world's wisdom'. Indeed many, if not all, the genuine oracles from the Sphinx and the Delphic Oracle, to the three witches in *Macbeth* appear to have been female. In Greek (pre-Hellenic) mythology, the chief deity of the Aegeans was—like that of many of the Asian cults—a female. She was called The Great Goddess, the Universal Mother, mistress of life, queen of death.

And to return to Plato's *Symposium*, but far in spirit and language from the clowning of Aristophanes, there is the solemn and fascinating story told by Socrates of a woman called Diotima of Mantineia who imparted to him the highest knowledge of the nature of love. Even the great Plato and his teacher Socrates were prepared to accord the highest knowledge to a woman!

In modern India the culture of the Hindu trains him to regard the mother as more worthy of reverence even than the father or the guru. A passage from 'Manu' may be translated thus:

From the point of view of reverence due, the guru is tenfold superior to a mere lecturer, a father a hundredfold to a guru, and a mother a thousandfold to a father.

153

The *ideal* of Indian womanhood is the same in the 1970s as in Vedic times, in other words the mark of the highest spirituality lies in a woman's attitude of undemanding love, compassion, modesty, and unselfishness. Needless to say, the modern Indian woman has had a hard struggle to realize her theoretical equality with men in ordinary everyday life, and faced, in the 1970s, with ever widening opportunities, she is often unsure of herself, bewildered by her new-found emancipation. This is because for fifteen hundred years the Indian woman was brought up as a model of Sita, the consort of Rama, whose life is described in the famous Hindu epic Ramayana. In the limited sphere in which she functioned, this ideal of womanhood was enough. But not any more. And it was largely due to the personal efforts of Sri Ramakrishna, his spiritual consort Sarada Devi, and Swami Vivekananda that the Indian woman of today has an ideal towards which she may evolve, and which is sufficient for her needs in the modern world.

This ideal is still spiritually based but may be aptly termed a *practical* spirituality. Swami Vivekananda, for all his forwardness of thinking, could not conceive of Indian womanhood without a background of religion. He believed that the Indian woman could and indeed must learn to live in a scientifically oriented world but not at the cost of her ancient heritage of spirituality. The ideal towards which to aim is a fusion of the two.

The Swami could not tolerate a way of life for any woman, or indeed for any man, which would tend to inhibit spiritual growth or the development of the intellect. So far as Indian women were concerned he knew that their greatest chance of realizing (and not just theorizing about) the Indian ideal of womanhood was to develop those feminine qualities of wisdom and sweetness and strength of character which are the hall-marks of Sri Sarada Devi, one of the most shining examples of Indian womanhood in modern times.

Chapter 15

THE USE AND MISUSE OF MIND

I think, therefore I am.

DESCARTES
Principes de la Philosophie

'WHY are we here?' One hears this asked so frequently that it is not unreasonable to infer that it is a standard question posed by thinking people the world over. It is a question to which the answer must inevitably be, 'We do not know.'

And indeed we do not and may not ever know because we lack the proper instrument for the task of finding out. No one can build a wall with pine needles or walk without limbs. In the same way we can say that Man cannot solve, to his satisfaction, the great Cosmic Riddle using the human mind as an instrument, because human thought is not the right one for such an undertaking. Certainly we can conjecture but we cannot *know* with any degree of certainty the answer to questions such as this.

Psychologists are of the opinion that the real purpose of the human intellect is the adjustment of man to the vicissitudes of life on earth. We are alive and must make the best of it each according to his particular temperament. It is a challenge to any thinking person and of itself can be a satisfactory goal towards which to aim. In so doing we can each play our part in adding to the store of human knowledge. Or to put it another way we can, if we decide to take up the challenge, wage our own unique battle against Man's huge ignorance. For that task the human intellect is an eminently suitable instrument.

So that if we make it our aim in life to live as fully as we can, without stopping to try to solve questions which to us are insoluble, we will waste none of our mental energy and will not fall prey to either pessimism, a bleak sense of futility or (most wasteful of all) boredom. It was the great artist, Rembrandt, who reputedly said that a man could find more beauty in his own village than could reasonably be enjoyed in one normal life span. There is no room for pessimism or boredom in such an attitude and goodness knows Rembrandt had as sad a life as one could imagine. But he never made the mistake of indulging in self-pity. He realized and accepted that life is not a rose garden and was prepared to face it as a fighting optimist.

If we look about us we can begin to understand what living fully really means. There is so much to see, to enjoy, to learn, and to experience. It is not necessary at first even to move from one's chair. I look at my two cats curled beside me as I sit at my desk. They are the colour of fresh cream. When I stop typing they look up and away into the middle distance, their eyes inscrutable. Their grace is something to please the eye, to charm the mind; their diverse temperaments give one pause. Why does the smaller one demand whatever he wants while the other (one of nature's gentlemen) quietly suggests he might perhaps have . . . Emotional blackmail? What else. Cats are clever, cleverer than we think. This afternoon I will go and buy some black paper and a white pencil and draw them in some of their incomparable attitudes. I used to draw a lot and wish I could draw better. Well now is the time to start practising. See what I mean? This is the kind of positive thinking that gets things done and prevents mental and physical inertia. It is not so easy to be bored. Above my head is a row of dictionaries. The blue one is Italian. If I learned a dozen new Italian words every day for three months and brushed up my Italian grammar I need never again ask for the libretto of a Verdi opera in English. . . .

Why waste time wondering why we are here? There is no law against spending your entire life wondering if you really must, but this is not living life fully. It is static and futile not to enjoy learning about the world in which we live, beginning with the things around us. If you think about it a man such as Rembrandt was not lacking in courage, and it is this very quality which is the keynote to the proper use of mind in the complex structure of modern civilization. The opposite is evasion which takes many forms such as abnormal inferiority complex, exaggerated self-deprecation, the various neuroses and (more dramatic but no less faint hearted) the death wish. Each may inhibit the individual to such a degree that he or she is unable to contribute to the common weal and, being ill-adjusted to his or her surroundings becomes, in effect, a social parasite. This kind of moral cowardice is a misuse of mind.

But how do we go about using the mind in a positive way? First we have to accept the fact that human beings actually *seek* experiences to feed their psychic life pattern in much the same way as they take in food to keep alive. And as we use our five physical senses to avoid food which might be poisonous we can, with time and practice, develop a similar mind-sense in order to examine each experience objectively before assimilating it. If an experience is appropriate to a *positive* life-pattern we can safely assimilate it. If not we are perfectly free to reject it.

It is possible to turn almost every experience to advantage by adjusting our viewpoint, but it is an established psychological fact that most people, far from learning from their experiences, actually go out of their way to create them to fit into the mosaic of their psychic life-patterns. This too is a misuse of mind, although entirely human and understandable. But it is far more profitable to adapt our way of life to fit our experiences than to distort our experiences to fit our established mind-pattern. The former carries with it the implication of broadening the mind to include new experiences.

A subjective attitude towards life's experiences is unalterably fixed, an objective one is flexible. In other words, a subjective person lives his life uneasily, trying to distort reality to match his preconceived ideas, while a well-adjusted person is able to expand his way of thought to meet reality. And so if we wish to be at ease with ourselves and our environment we must try to cultivate flexibility of mind. The more flexible we are, the more varied and purposeful our life experiences will be, leaving us no time for boredom or to ponder such unanswerable questions as 'Why are we here?'

Certain other negative or unsocial behaviour patterns betray the absence of any real purpose in, and affirmation of, life. For such behaviour patterns we can use the umbrella term neuroses. These are not diseases but negative attitudes towards life and its problems, the common denominator of which is a refusal to accept social responsibility. To the victim of a neurosis the everyday tasks and obligations of life assume a difficulty so grossly out of proportion to the facts that the neurotic is compelled to invent all manner of alibis as a substitute for their performance. It is common for neurotics to protest 'I would be able to work if only . . .' or 'I would get married if only . . .', or 'I would have more time to practise the piano if only . . .'. In all instances the neurotic evades responsibility and the reasons for this are legion and often complex, even bizarre. But it is generally agreed that in each case it is possible to detect an underlying sense of inferiority and a consequent inability to meet the obligations of life.

One then needs to ask what causes a sense of inferiority, and can it be alleviated? It is fairly obvious that any form of real or imagined physical disability is a contributory factor. But in many cases the inferiority complex acts as a spur to people of strong mettle or outstanding ability. Napoleon was below average height, Beethoven was deaf, Pitt was abnormally thin, Chopin was frail in health, Toulouse-Lautrec was deformed—the list is long and varied. Apropos of this I would mention in passing that a book written in 1942, *The Varieties of Temperament* by W. H. Sheldon, contains the intriguing theory that neurosis can be, and often is, caused by the futile efforts of people to become something other than that to which their physical structure would naturally incline them. It is suggested that physique and character are closely related although much research remains to be done to substantiate this hypothesis.

It is important to know that the complexity of Man's psychic structure and his long initial period of helplessness render inevitable the conflicts which result in neurosis, and also that there does not exist any person who is not, or has not at some time been neurotic to some degree. But there is a difference between the so-called normal person and one who is sufficiently at the mercy of inner disharmony to need psychiatric help, though I stress that this difference is one of degree and not of kind. The existence of even a severe degree of neurosis in no way precludes worldly or intellectual achievement and it is a pyschological fact that certain types of outstanding success cannot in fact be achieved at all without a compulsive power drive which would, by any standards, be regarded by psychiatrists as pathological.

Conversely the presence of a severe degree of neurosis in no way guarantees worldly success. There are severely neurotic people who achieve success and those whose lives are almost completely crippled by their inner conflicts. Similarly there are both successful people and social drop-outs who would be classed as normal by psychiatrists. But an analytical inquiry into the inter-personal relationships of so-called neurotic people would always reveal a lack of emotional maturity which one can say requires that the personality remain recognizably the same under varying circumstances. How the individual responds to the presence of neurosis determines the degree of success he would be likely to achieve.

Some people are neurotic to such a degree that their personalities are completely stunted. This is due to conflict between the essentially self-regulating psyche and the fear of being inadequate and therefore of not being accepted by one's fellows. The extent to which the emotionally developing child is able to understand and accept his own nature determines the degree of neurosis later in life. Unfortunately it is difficult to determine the differing psychological requirements and reactions of each individual child until the first five years are over, by which time it is too late. But then no child ever developes without conflict because some deviation from its own essential nature is inevitable. The child has to be 'good', which means he has to conform to what his parents insist is good, and if he is 'bad' the child will soon learn to fear that his parents will withdraw their love and protection, a notion which is intolerable to any child. And so the effort to conform, in conflict with his own natural inclinations, results inevitably in some degree of frustration and tension. The most we can hope for in the child/parent relationship is that it will go reasonably well so that by the time the child reaches adulthood he will have discovered his own real nature and accepted it. If the parents are sufficiently adult themselves to welcome the child's differentiation from themselves the child will feel secure in their love and protection. But if the child is prevented from accepting his own nature the result will almost certainly be a noticeable degree of neurosis, which is the device of the psyche for the evasion of responsibility.

Certain other devices such as egoism, vanity and conceit, are used for various purposes by people with a sense of inferiority or those who have not achieved sufficient confidence, in order to avoid making any contribution to the welfare of society in general or assuming social responsibilities. These people are still emotional infants and this again is a misuse of mind because a full life implies a flexible variety in our experiences and actions, and character is built up by exposure to these. Yoga philosophy reiterates that the selfishness and private logic of the egoist is in opposition to all the laws of common sense.

The completely selfless person has yet to be born and this must be understood by all students of Yoga. An intelligent approach to this fact is to accept that it is futile to try to eliminate completely all vanity, egoism, selfishness and conceit from the character because even were it possible, it would lead to a repulsive sanctimoniousness. So moderation is the operative and common sense word. Humility can so easily become a vice if it is made the chief life-activity, although in moderation it is an undisputed virtue. But students of Yoga are always warned that absolutely no virtue is of sufficient importance to deserve the *total* involvement of our mental energies.

What then can one do if egoism, vanity and conceit are inherent in the character of every human being? How does Yogic common sense deal with this problem? Quite simply, one does not engage in a futile struggle with undesirable character traits but diverts them into socially useful channels, an activity which is perfectly feasible. Like both egoism and vanity, a potential socially useful force is ambition. Although wealth and prestige may be the end products they do not of themselves bring inner peace of mind or resolve conflicts. If the individual is entirely selfish in his ambition and demands a degree of security beyond the confines of normal human needs, he will reap little in terms of social popularity which is only to be found in proportion to the amount of understanding, patience and philanthropy which the individual feels and displays towards his fellow men.

No one can be in a state of inner harmony in work which centres exclusively around the satisfaction of his own immediate needs. It would be infinitely more satisfying if everyone could commit himself to a programme of social activity, if each person's centre of gravity could move to some social concern outside his own person. In this way it would be possible to learn at first hand the value of surrendering the ego to the service of one's fellow men. Two quotations, one from the Gita, one from Schopenhauer, illustrate this.

That man who lives devoid of longing, abandoning all desires, without the sense of 'I' and 'mine', he attains to peace.

Bhagavad Gita II

Every violent exhibition of will is commonplace and vulgar; in other words, it reduces us to the level of the species, and makes us a mere type and example of it.

SCHOPENHAUER

Yoga students are reminded by their teachers that they should try to make it one of their primary aims to increase their humanity by any means available to them which their ingenuity can invent. The truly mature and socially integrated person can always find the time to stop and listen to the affairs and woes of his fellow beings. It is only the self-centred and the neurotic who cannot find the time for other people.

Those who would increase their humanity should endeavour to expand their occupational interests and social horizons, in other words put Karma Yoga into practice. And if work is a source of personal expansion the best kind of work is an occupation which affords some measure of compensation for some inferiority feeling in terms of social usefulness. And each person we meet affords us an opportunity for constructive social behaviour.

Each one of us is endowed with a unique personality which seeks its own realization, and the cut and thrust of enduring inter-personal relationships affords us a chance of drawing nearer to this goal. This innate drive towards self-realization is an instinctive force which impels the individual towards an increasingly complete realization and expression of his potentialities.

One must point out that self-realization does not imply a disregard of individual differences. People vary in countless ways and the goal to aim for is a satisfactory relationship between the world and one-self according to our diverse interests, needs, and abilities. Man is a social animal and the non-acceptance of this basic fact is a misuse of mind. Man's characteristic pattern of coping with the difficulties of existence has always, so far as we can deduce, been the formation of social groups. An isolated human being could maintain life and sanity only by means of knowledge gained from other human beings. The social community, whether it be a family, clan, tribe, race or nation, is an essential of human life. We can say then that one way to use the mind correctly is first and foremost to be a member of some kind of group. In this way each individual gains security as nearly as any being possibly can. That person who, most completely and effectively utilizes the bonds which link him to his fellows is most secure in his humanity. Tolstoy, in a letter to Gandhi, had this to say:

Love, which is the striving for the union of human souls and the activity derived from it, is the highest and only law of human life, and in the depth of his soul every human being feels and knows this. He knows this until he is entangled by the false teachings of the world.

Two further essential ingredients are necessary to the correct use of mind, namely knowledge and organization. This perhaps requires a word of explanation. Simply if one has no knowledge of a subject there is no starting point for thought, but on the other hand all the knowledge in the world would be of little use without the organization of those thoughts. The first example of this that comes to mind is something I once experienced. Imagine that someone borrows your typewriter or you send it away for cleaning and it is returned with the carriage locked. How many people use their typewriters and never use the carriage lock. As a matter of fact it is not strictly necessary to do so unless the machine is to be carried. So what do you do if you do not know how to release the carriage? Most people would arbitrarily move every lever and button until by chance they happened upon the right one. This could be, and usually is, time-wasting and a complete misuse of mind. A much more logical and efficient way to solve this simple problem is to examine the machine, disregard all the keys, buttons, levers etc. of which you actually know the function which reduces the numbers of possible right ones to a minimum. Then look for others systematically, move each one and you will eventually release the carriage. One could argue that this, too, could take time. Granted, but at least you are using your mind logically, and the more practice you get the more instinctive the habit will become. Yoga and logic are blood brothers and one of the most formidable enemies of logical thought is *prejudice*.

This is a problem with which Yoga teachers have grappled for centuries. The student is first urged to realize that man was a victim of his emotions—fear, pleasure, anger, frustration etc.—long before he was able to think, but although these emotions are too deep-seated to be disregarded, they do cause us to be suggestible and prejudiced, and distort our thinking. My own teacher used to reiterate that prejudgement is a common human failing but that we must try to be aware of when we prejudge and endeavour to break the habit. Judges would likely confess that it is difficult enough to pass judgement when one is in possession of all, or nearly all, the relevant facts. How much more difficult would be a judgement when one possessed few or no facts at all. The result is downright injustice, which is exactly what prejudice is.

Another form of prejudice is thinking in extremes. For example, if a man sees a woman driver behaving foolishly he is more than likely to say to himself, 'Women are terrible drivers.' If a woman tries on a hat and it doesn't suit her she might afterwards happily tell her friends, 'I don't wear hats, they don't suit me.' These two examples are comparatively harmless but what of the person who marries and afterwards is compelled to seek a divorce. To say, 'I will not marry again. Women (or men) are impossible' is a prejudgement which can deprive an individual of an experience which can be the most rewarding and satisfying in adult life.

There is no complete answer to the bad habit of prejudging but the realization that we are all, to some extent prejudiced and suggestible, that we are prey to our emotions and tend to find some form of rationalization for our motives should, up to a point, lead to more positive and effective thought. And the habit of logical and effective thought can, in time, dispel some if not all our prejudices. At least let us recognize that the problem does exist.

Another step on the road to the correct use of mind is to try to discard some of our defective thought patterns. It is again entirely commonplace for one's thought to be directed along certain lines for no other reason than that they have been so directed all one's life. But the fact of thinking that this or that is a fact does not make it so. Too many people believe things which are entirely fallacious, without giving them the slightest thought. Take any cliché: an hour's sleep before midnight is better than two hours after; black cats are lucky; thirteen is unlucky; always serve red wine with meat and white wine with fish (gourmets will tell you this is a fallacy). But these old worn-out phrases are mindlessly believed by the majority. And so the next time someone hands you a cliché stop and think before accepting it. By all means accept it if it is common sense, but not otherwise. In fact we have constantly to question everything, to take nothing on its face value if we are to cultivate the correct use of mind.

Another pitfall is the habit of being dogmatic and always believing you are in the right. Apart from being intensely irritating to the people with whom you live or work, the dogmatic person is so rigid in his thinking that there is no room for growth in his mental make-up. Now and again it is healthy and sensible to check those dearly held convictions to see if they are still valid. If they are, well and good. If they are not, at least have the courage to discard them.

Curiosity is one of the mainsprings of the correct use of mind and yet it is astonishing how many people have an almost total lack of curiosity. We all know people who take life as it comes and simply ignore anything they do not understand. One of the greatest services Yoga does to human thought is to train its students to take a healthy interest in anything new or strange and to try to understand, accept, and assimilate it. Think of what the world's music would be like if composers such as Bach, Handel, Mozart and Beethoven had not wondered about and experimented with the discord, or Wagner with the modulation, or Stravinsky with jazz idioms. And what would great painting have been like if Manet had simply listened to other artists saying, 'Do not use black, it makes a hole in the painting', and not experimented with it to see what he could do. And if the great French impressionists had not been curious about the effects of light on water and on solid objects. Or if the great scientific inventors had not been curious about the physical world and the effects of one substance upon another.

If curiosity is one of the mainsprings in the correct use of mind, the opposite effect is produced by procrastination which implies a lack of real interest, and a state of indecision. At times procrastination can be almost pathological, such as when a person has a positive phobia about making decisions in case the wrong one is made or the result be failure. And it is a psychological fact that the longer one takes in coming to a decision the more difficult it becomes, and the fact of putting off making a decision implies that one is avoiding the issue. As I have said, a common device is for people to say, 'I will do this and that when the right time comes', or 'I will marry when the right man/woman appears on the scene'. People with this attitude towards making decisions are positively courting lost opportunities. The time to start something is *now*, unless circumstances positively preclude it. For those who suffer from a fear of failure (and very many people do have this problem) it helps to remember that every occasion which affords us an opportunity to learn something adds strength to the personality and increases our capacity to meet, understand and solve new problems.

And on the subject of problems, it will save a lot of time and mental fatigue if you practise taking a common sense approach to the minor problems which beset us in our day to day life. For instance if you dread going to the dentist you can cut down the misery of it all by deciding to visit him regularly every six months. In this way there will be no long and painful sessions, and anything needing to be done will be a minor matter. If you worry about losing your job because you cannot get up in the morning buy a really sadistic alarm clock, set it each night and place it at the opposite side of the room from your bed. You will have to get out of bed to silence it (of course you will have to exercise will power to stop yourself from

164

crawling back into bed). The small nagging worries of everyday life *can* get in your hair if you let them. But I can hear some of my readers saying 'Yes, but I am a worrier by nature so what can I do about it?' There is at least one device which I learned from my own teacher. 'Ask yourself', she used to say, 'what is the very worst thing that can happen if this and that happens?' For instance, did you leave the light on when you left home, did you turn out the oven, did you lock the back door, your car door, the garage door and so on? And if it turns out that you forgot, well now what is the worst thing that can happen? A slightly larger electricity bill, a burnt offering, is it a calamity? Yes, you will say, but what if it is a burglary? I can assure you that whichever door you forgot to lock, you will never forget to lock it again! And if you own anything valuable, it is common sense to insure it. That would be another worry you could dismiss from your mind, leaving you that much more time to use it properly. It has been said that compared with what we ought to be we are only half awake. We use only a small fraction of our mental resources. Perhaps at this stage in human evolution it is not possible to utilize one hundred per cent of all our resources, but if we make the effort to improve our mental efficiency, we can at least derive some satisfaction from the fact that we are using our minds properly.

Chapter 16

WHICH YOGA IS YOURS?

Love will find its way
Through paths where wolves would fear to prey.
BYRON *The Giaour*

YOU HAVE reached the last chapter of my book and perhaps the whole subject of Yoga now intrigues you. So naturally you might wish to try it for yourself. But how do you begin? *Where* do you begin? And most important of all, as you now know there are four Yogas, which is the right one for you?

Consider your overall life-pattern and your basic character type. Have you got everything you want and if not, what is it you do want? How much time are you able and prepared to give to the study of Yoga? Can it help you? Do you think you need it at all?

Everyone has problems. Let us consider yours. One of the primary curses of our modern industrial environment is nervous tension. This brings in its wake any or all of the following symptoms: insomnia, the inability to relax, nameless fears, anxieties and worries, headaches, irritability, depression, and every neurosis in the book. It can also cause overweight. How? Any Yoga teacher or psychologist can tell you how people turn to food for comfort when they feel 'down'. Many a person who suffers from nervous tension is a compulsive eater. I come across it all the time among my own pupils. Any Yoga teacher can spot the symptoms half a mile away. Fortunately it is an easy problem to cure—I wish some of the others were half so easy!

Physical problems are legion in our modern so-called civilized society, mental problems perhaps even more so. The latter I intend to discuss in detail in my next book, so here I will confine myself to physical ailments. No Yoga teacher will mind if you go to him or her and say, 'I do not feel well, I have this and that. Can you do something about it?' If that is all you want from Yoga then your best plan is to study Hatha Yoga and leave it at that. My first book on Yoga, *Yoga and Your Health*, is all about Hatha Yoga and how it can cure physical ailments of all kinds.

I always think of Hatha Yoga as the 'little brother' of Raja Yoga, one of the four main Yogas. Hatha Yoga is mainly concerned with posture, breathing, diet, and the control of the body. Raja Yoga, often called the 'Royal Yoga' is the study of control of the mind. Even without aspiring to Raja Yoga, the student of Hatha will find his physical health improved beyond all belief. This is by no means to be despised, although I have met many so-called 'spiritual' types who will have nothing to do with Hatha Yoga because its province is mainly the physical body. I do not find any logic in this kind of attitude. How can a person begin to control his mind if he is plagued by indigestion, a splitting headache, or any other physical discomfort? To my way of thinking it is nonsense even to try.

Basically Hatha Yoga *is* a means to an end. It is a preliminary to the study of Raja Yoga, which is extremely difficult and requires a lot of patience and practice, so much in fact that most people find it beyond their capabilities. Yoga teachers know this perfectly well, and think no less of their pupils if they ask to be taught Hatha Yoga and no more.

So if you are the active, athletic type, or if you continually feel in a state of 'sub-health', then your Yoga is Hatha. It is by far the most popular form of Yoga in the Western world. Indeed most people think it is the *only* Yoga. I would be glad if some of the fallacies about Yoga would only stop there. But no! Uninformed people often speak of Yoga as some dark, esoteric practice of magical rites for attaining miraculous powers—something like Black Magic you could say. If this were so could I, could *anyone* write a book called *Common Sense About Yoga*? Is there anyone who could write a sensible book called *Common Sense About Black Magic*?

Yoga is based on logic and on human psychology. If you study it for long enough it gives you an incredible insight into other people. Yoga teachers have this insight and it often stuns their pupils. It is possible to diagnose a pupil's problem and know what his needs are as he walks through the door, but there is no more magic to it than a medical specialist displays if he can, and some doctors certainly can, diagnose a patient's ailments as he walks through the door. Some doctors are good diagnosticians. It is not guesswork, it is a gift. Yoga teachers are good diagnosticians from years of practice in dealing with human beings, from years of study of psychology, from logic and from minute observance of other people. It is easy when you know how. There is no magic in it.

There is a Yoga in accordance with each person's natural tendencies, abilities and inclinations. There are four main Yogas, starting with Raja (with Hatha Yoga as its preliminary), and Karma Yoga to which I have devoted a whole chapter. What of the other two, Bhakti Yoga and Jnana Yoga? Let us deal with Bhakti Yoga first. The central principle of Bhakti Yoga is to learn the various feelings and emotions in the human mind, and to know that they are not wrong in themselves. But they do have to be controlled, otherwise they themselves will take control. So ask yourself whether or not you prefer to use your intuition rather than your reason. Do you believe that love, rather than achievement, is the great ennobling influence in life? Are you naturally religious? Are you self-sacrificing? If you can answer 'yes' to these questions then you have found your natural Yoga. It is Bhakti.

It has one great advantage and one great disadvantage. It is, without doubt, the easiest of the Yogas if you happen to be inclined that way. In fact if you are a natural Bhakti, you will find Bhakti Yoga is part of your own nature, and because of this it will make far fewer demands upon you than would the study of one of the other Yogas. Its disadvantage is that it can sometimes degenerate into fanaticism. In other words, you are right and everyone else is wrong. That is not Yoga. If you can only love your own ideal by hating every other ideal, that is not Yoga, it is fanaticism. Sri Ramakrishna used to say, 'As many faiths, so many paths.' *That* is Yoga.

Bhakti Yoga lays on its followers the imperative command not to hate or deny or despise any other human being, either for his method of worship or for the way he chooses to conduct his life. The question of the food he eats has always been a vital one with the Bhakti. This too can degenerate into fanaticism. So I would suggest to the beginner that he read the Bhagavad Gita and pay particular attention to what is said about food and follow the instructions. In this way he can avoid the pitfall of what is often referred to as 'driving religion into the kitchen'!

Bhakti Yoga involves keeping the body scrupulously clean and eating pure foods. These two matters are easy. But then we come to cleanliness of mind and character, and this is where the hardest work comes in. There is a list of qualities given by Ramanuja, a famous saint and philosopher of southern India, which reads as follows:

'Truthfulness, sincerity, selfless good deeds, non-injury to others by thought, word or deed, not coveting that which another person owns, complete absence of vanity and complete absence of vengefulness and jealousy.'

Another attribute of the true Bhakti is cheerfulness. That might sound strange to our Western minds because we tend to think of religious people as long-faced and devoid of humour. Actually it is not true—even in the West—but it is the general supposition. In Yoga it is said that the cheerful mind is better equipped to persevere and hack its way through a jungle of difficulties than one which makes heavy going of the mental disciplines involved. But Yoga and moderation are first cousins, so at the same time excessive levity or mirth is frowned upon, because it fritters away mental energy. The ideal state of mind at which to aim in Bhakti Yoga is one of equilibrium.

This is by no means all there is to Bhakti Yoga, but it will give my readers a general idea as to the kind of person who is suited to practise it rather than the other Yogas. Basically it suits the religious, contemplative type of person, and the more practical types tend to leave it alone. In fact the people who are essentially practical by nature and who like to mix with other people are naturally suited to Karma Yoga.

And what of the fourth Yoga, Jnana? It does not come last by any means—all four Yogas are equal and in fact they tend to overlap. I merely left Jnana Yoga to the last because it is such a huge subject. Actually it needs a whole chapter to itself—a whole book even, but I do not feel that the Western world is ready for Jnana Yoga yet. I gave a whole chapter to Karma Yoga because it is both the most practical of the four Yogas and also the most extrovert, and therefore it seems to me to be ideally suited to our modern times, and when it becomes better known in the West it may well equal Hatha Yoga in popularity. We shall have to see.

So what of Jnana Yoga? This is the Yoga of the intellect, of discrimination, and of reasoning. It is the Yoga of analysis and the natural sciences. Jnana Yoga could be summed up as the heightening of our consciousness through study and mental analysis. It is suited to people who like to reason, who like to study, who love knowledge for its own sake. It is the Yoga of the intellectual, and because the overwhelming majority of people do not like to use their brains, to pile up knowledge for its own sake, most people would find Jnana

Yoga very hard going indeed.

But for those people to whom it might make a strong appeal I will elaborate a little. It examines basic philosophical questions such as the real nature of man, ethics, immortality, freedom and spiritual bondage, and the discrimination between illusion and reality. It examines psychology, and the dualistic conception of good and evil: are they two separate entities or are they diverse manifestations of one and the same fact? It examines the sciences, it examines cause and effect. As I said, it is a huge subject, and a fascinating one. If you like to know *things*, if you cannot rest until you understand something, then this is your Yoga.

There, then, are the four principal Yogas. You will know best which one most appeals to you—but do remember that they are, as it were, all paths up the same mountain at the summit of which is Self-Awareness. Yoga awaits your interest, your inspection, your first hesitant experiments. It is here, it has always been here, it is yours for the taking. But to practicalities. Let us suppose you have chosen your particular Yoga, where do you go from there?

Try to find a teacher. They are thin on the ground in the West but some people are lucky enough to find one. This is the easiest way to learn Yoga, from someone who has been studying it for years. But supposing you are not lucky enough to find a teacher, what then? Read an English translation of the Bhagavad Gita—after all why not go to the fountain-head if you want to learn something? The Gita contains all the fundamental principles of Yogic philosophy. It is a beautiful book but like all great literature it requires study. You would not read Plato or Aristotle through once and throw them aside, would you? If you can read them at all, and read the Gita through to the end, does it not mean that you are searching for something? You may not be aware of what that something is, in fact you may not be aware that you are searching at all. So learn to watch what you do, what you read, the kind of people with whom you choose to mix. This is a great help in knowing yourself and that is Yoga too.

In a whole library of books which one do you pick up? You have to be honest with yourself. You may pick up a book on philosophy or on any other subject which requires you to think, and think hard —you can pick up the book but if it is not in your nature to ponder on high principles you will not be able to fool yourself because you will not be able to read it. It is the same with the Bhagavad Gita.

Some people pick it up and cannot put it down. Others cannot read it. So your very first lesson in Yoga is to try to be honest with yourself and remember that in no way can you change your own basic nature. That is not the aim of Yoga, nor does it make you into a saint. It deepens insight, it will make you into a more understanding person, a more compassionate and peaceful one. If you can learn to be at peace with yourself you will be at peace with everything and everyone else, so you will certainly be a happier person.

Yoga is hard work but then so is everything else worthwhile. Having chosen your particular path it may at times appear to be too rocky and you may feel you cannot go on. If this happens, and it often does, remember the words of the Gita:

With the sword of the understanding of thyself thou shalt rend asunder in thy heart every doubt arising from ignorance, and thou shalt achieve thy permanence in Yoga.